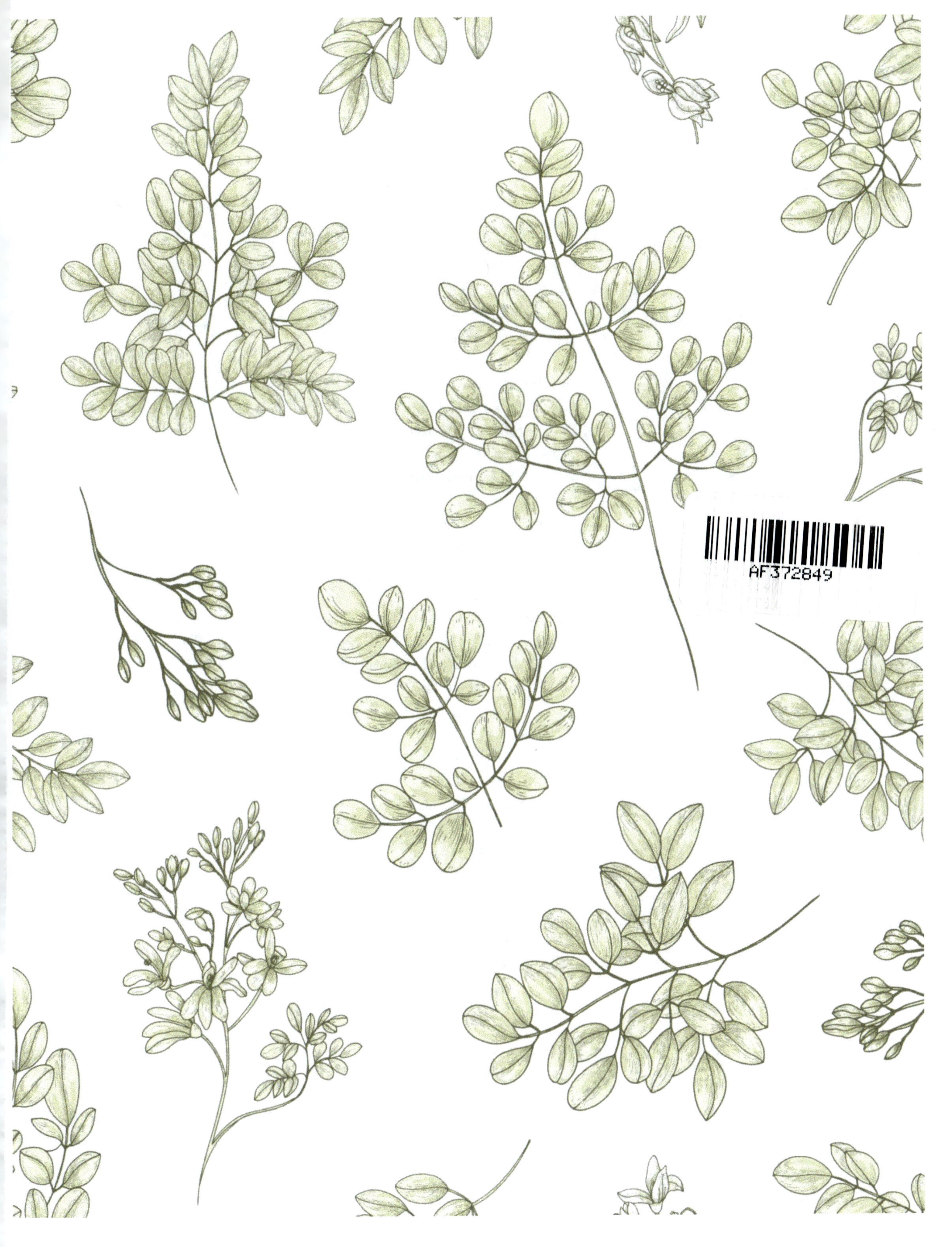
AF372849

Project Manager Yee MC
Editor Mimi Ngu
Art Director SY Hoo
Photographers Kelly Mohd Nor,
Wah Fahmy Redzuan

Perpustakaan Negara Malaysia
Cataloguing-in-Publication Data

Published by
Mohana Rosie Gill Nee M R Dutt
moringalicious: FOR HEALTHY LIVING,
LONGEVITY, AND WELLNESS/Mohana Gill
Address
48, Jalan Tanjong,
46000 Petaling Jaya,
Selangor

ISBN-978-629-98780-0-1
1. Cooking, Malaysian.
2. Cookbooks.
3. Recipes.
I. Title.

Printed in Malaysia by
Precision Offset Solutions
Level 2, No. 2,
Jalan Anggerik Vanilla,
Kota Kemuning,
40460 Shah Alam,
Selangor

MORINGALICIOUS

For Healthy Living, Longevity, and Wellness

MOHANA GILL

**Dedicated to my mother,
Leela Dutt.**

*She was always beautifully dressed in
exquisite, self-embroidered sarees,
and she wore flowers in her hair.*

*She was a wildflower of Burma,
fearless and always ready to conquer rough soils.*

She was a woman ahead of her time.

She was my mother, Leela.

---

*"Every time I think about quitting something,
I just remember my mother and the fact that
if she didn't show her strength to keep going, then I wouldn't be alive.
And it makes me feel like a coward for even thinking of giving up"*
- Michael Phelps

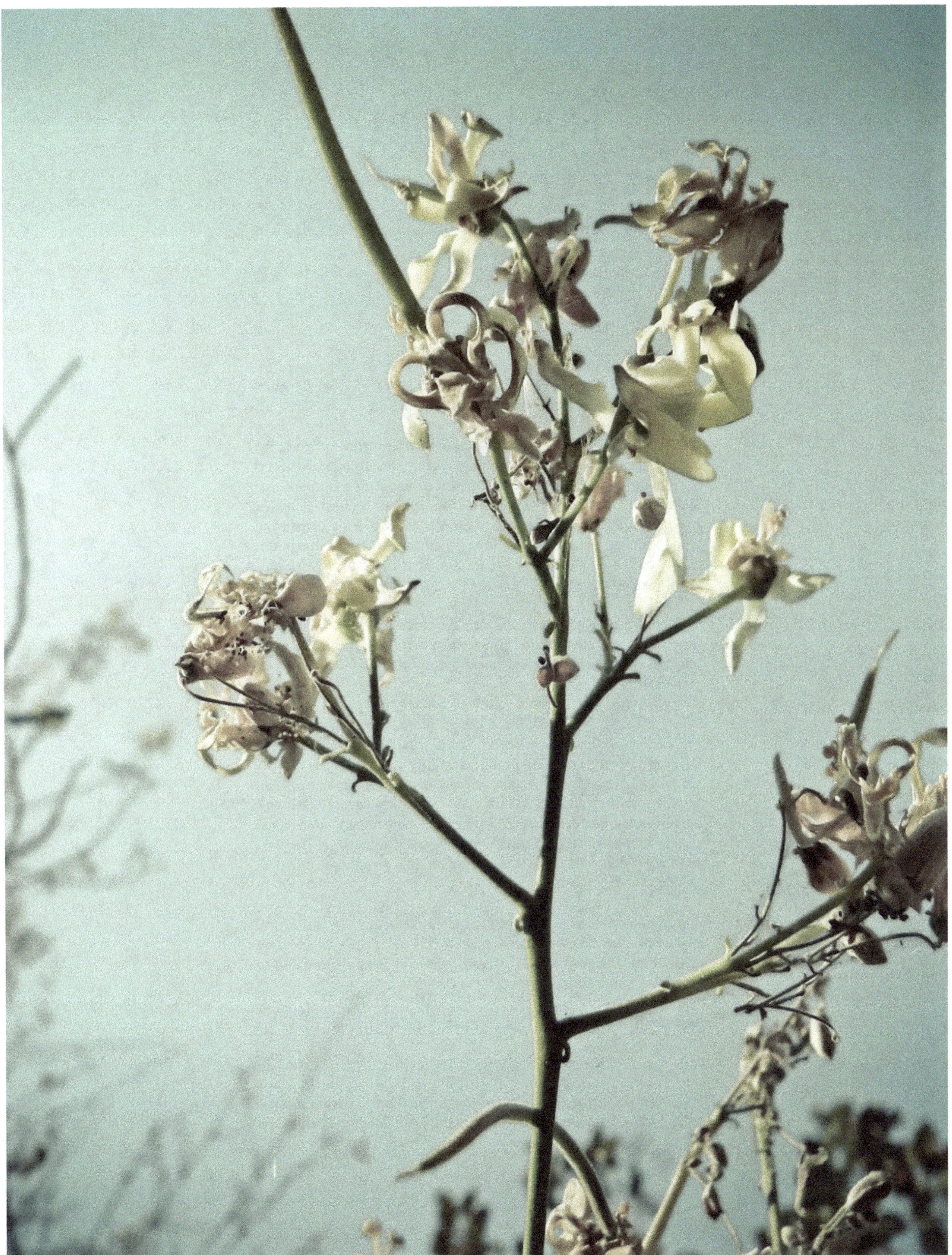

FOREWORD

I am honoured to be given this opportunity to write the foreword for *Moringalicious: For Healthy Living, Longevity, and Wellness* by multi award-winning and distinguished author Mohana Gill.

I am very happy that I am a part of this recipe book as I truly believe in the benefits of moringa—I even have a moringa tree growing in the backyard of my house in Petaling Jaya! Having savoured some of the recipes featured in this book, I look forward to trying my hands at learning them all so that I, too, can bring the many benefits of the Miracle Tree to my kitchen and onto the dining table, to share with my family and friends. Through this book, you can do the same for your loved ones and spread the health-giving goodness of moringa.

With her sharp culinary skills and meticulous attention to detail, Mohana has come up with more than 60 ways to enjoy moringa in dishes that cover international cuisines, and everything from appetisers to main course and even desserts.

When Mohana speaks of the moringa dishes she enjoys cooking, her passion is palpable—infectious, even—especially given the close connection to her childhood in Burma and the beautiful memories she shared with her mother. The transcendence of love from mother to child is evident in this book, which couldn't have come at a better time. In this post-pandemic world, health and wellness are more important now than ever, and the spotlight is on natural remedies such as moringa. The good news is, we don't need to look far as the moringa tree can be found all around us and grows easily.

Through *Moringalicious*, Mohana has crafted a legacy of wisdom, advice, health tips, and delectable recipes aimed at nourishing present and future generations. This book is also a testament to her lifelong dedication to promoting healthy living, longevity, and wellness.

That is why I truly believe that *Moringalicious* is Malaysia's gift to the world.

From the desk of **YAM Tengku Puteri Nor Zehan Binti Almarhum Sultan Salahuddin Abdul Aziz Shah Alhaj Tengku Puan Panglima Perlis**

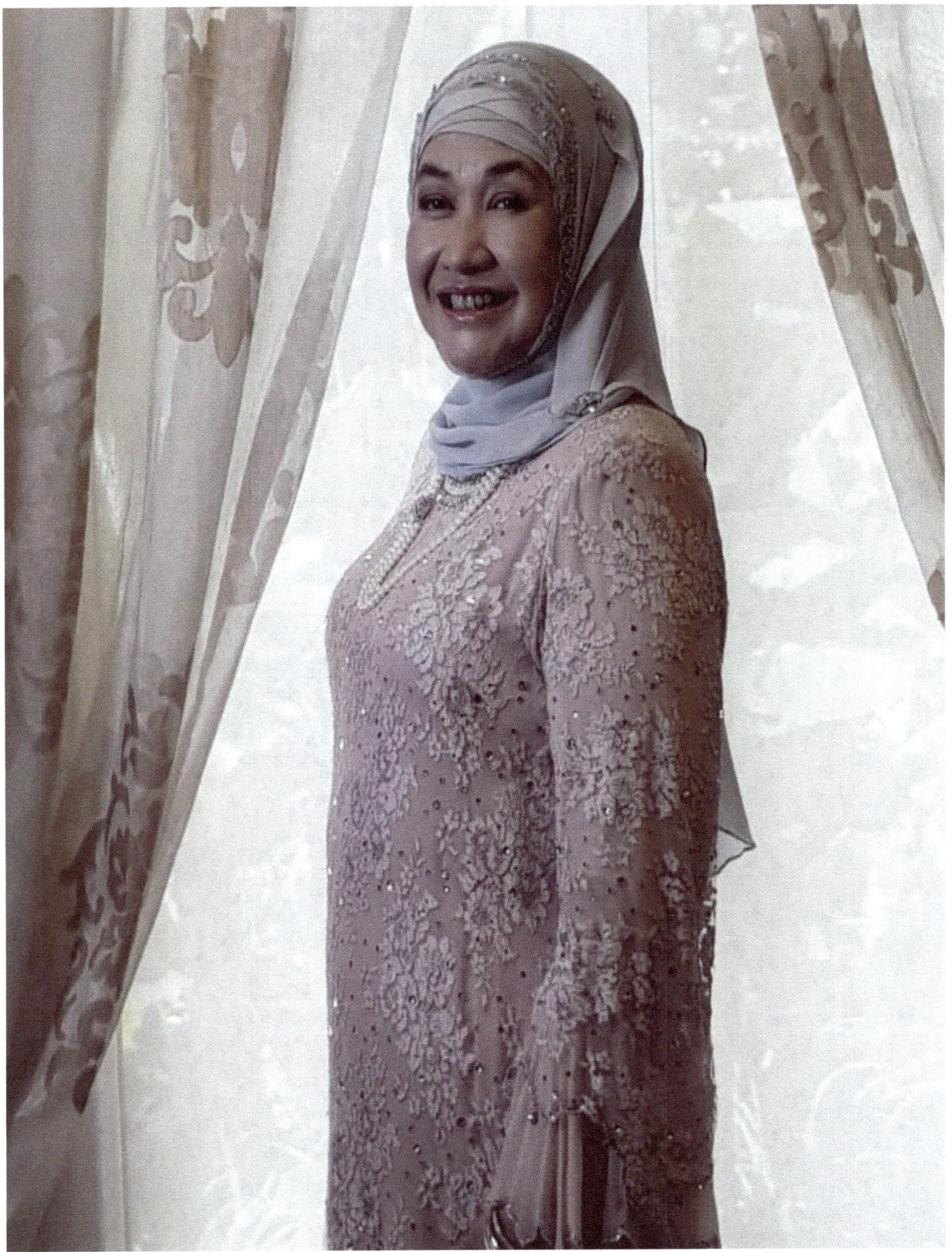

AUTHOR'S NOTE

As you hold this cookbook in your hands, you are stepping into my culinary journey that began in the heart of Burma (now Myanmar), where I was born and raised.

Growing up, the moringa tree was a familiar sight for me as it grew abundantly all around. At home, it featured regularly on our dining table as my mother, Leela, would whip up a wonderful array of dishes that starred every part of the amazing Tree of Life—from its delicate flowers to the soft leaves and drumsticks encasing that wonderful gelatinous flesh within. I could never resist the temptation to sneak into the kitchen whenever my mother prepared one of her moringa-infused dishes and watch her lovingly craft a meal from scratch. In my young mind, cooking was very much like magic: simple, fresh, everyday ingredients were transformed into a myriad aromas, colours, flavours, and textures that whet the appetite, satiated every tastebud, and left lingering memories.

Little did I know then that those cherished moments would cast a lifelong spell on me, shaping my passion for cooking and inspiring my life journey from Burma to Malaysia, which became my home after I got married. When I first moved to Kuala Lumpur, everything felt strange and unfamiliar, but I found solace in the familiar sight of the moringa trees that grow commonly here too. It was my connection to home; it warmed my heart to know that I could share a taste of my childhood with my own family and nourish them with all the goodness of moringa.

The recipes in this book are a culmination of decades of shared joys—some passed down by my mother and others discovered through camaraderie in the kitchen with exceptional women, including my dear Filipino helpers, Lyn and Christine. Every dish is a symphony of garden-fresh leaves, dainty flowers, and robust drumsticks, all handpicked from the moringa trees that thrive in my very own garden. It truly is a garden-to-table odyssey that you'll embark on as you flip through the pages. Every recipe is a tribute to the nourishing essence of moringa, combining wholesome ingredients and heartfelt techniques to create dishes suitable for all ages.

As a cookbook author, I have always implored the importance of healthy living, longevity, and wellness, and the moringa is the epitome of that. You can easily grow moringa in your home garden, as I have. It requires little attention yet flourish beautifully. Imagine if countries around the world make it a priority to plant moringa trees all around, then people can easily obtain nutritious food everywhere! I truly believe that the moringa is one of God's greatest gifts to mankind and in creating *Moringalicious*, I envision it as Malaysia's gift to the world.

May *Moringalicious* inspire you to create, indulge, and savour the traditions and flavours that have shaped my life, one moringa-infused dish at a time.

From my kitchen to yours,

Mohana Gill

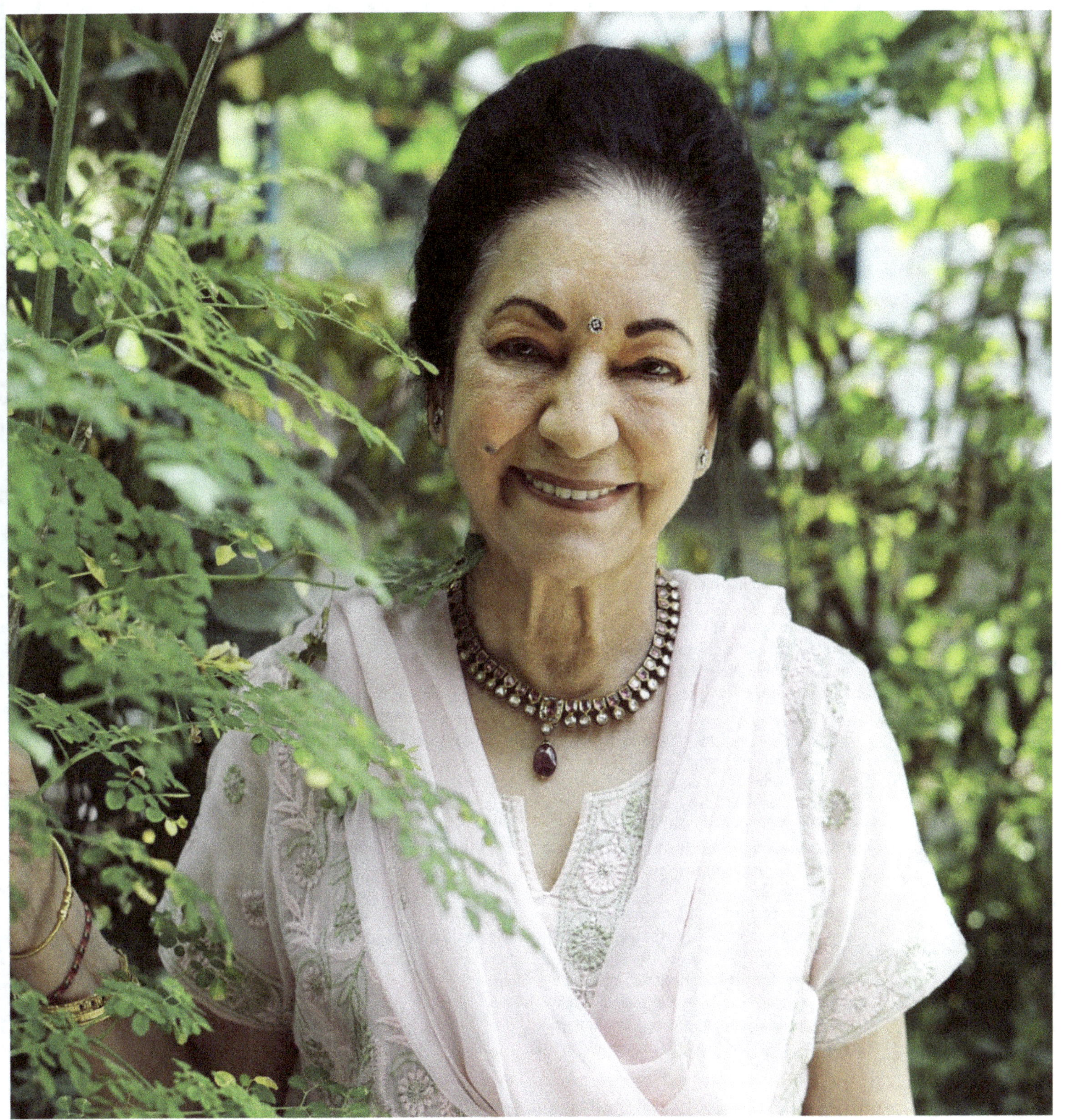

"My mission in life is not merely to survive, but to thrive,
and to do so with some passsion, some compassion,
some humour, and some style"
- Maya Angelou

A TALE OF THE MORINGA TREE

This was a story that my mother, Leela,
often told of World War I in Burma.

There was a beautiful moringa tree that grew in front of the house that Leela and her family lived. The tree was in full bloom; its delicate white flowers were not only beautiful and edible, they were delicious and had a lot of health properties.

During the war, all universities in Rangoon (now Yangon) were closed and the students returned to their homes. Leela had a very good friend who had two daughters studying medicine at the University of Rangoon. Both the girls had returned home to be with their parents. Leela invited her friend and the two girls to tea. She admired the two girls and hoped that one day, her children would also go to university and study medicine like the girls.

When her friend and daughters saw the moringa tree, they were intrigued. They wanted to have some of the moringa flowers and Leela promised them that she would get them some.

A little boy of about 11 or 12 years was asked to come and help pluck the flowers. He climbed up on the tree and shook the branches while the girls and Leela's daughters picked them up off the ground below. Now, the branches of the moringa tree were quite brittle. Suddenly, one of them gave way under the boy's weight and he went tumbling down! Fortunately, it wasn't a very high branch and he was barely hurt. But unfortunately, he did fall onto the legs of one of Leela's daughters—the second, Veena—and broke her leg!

Panic ensued; Veena was rushed to the hospital and had to be admitted and operated on. After the surgery, she couldn't bend her leg as it had to be placed in a cast. That meant she couldn't walk properly either, which caused her parents to worry. The days passed by anxiously. Finally, after a week, Veena's cast could be removed and her leg had healed well enough for her to bend it. She was able to walk properly again—which was lucky timing, as the air raids began that very day. If Veena's leg was still in a cast, she would have needed to be carried to the trenches!

"In three words,
I can sum up everything
I've learned about life: it goes on"
- Robert Frost

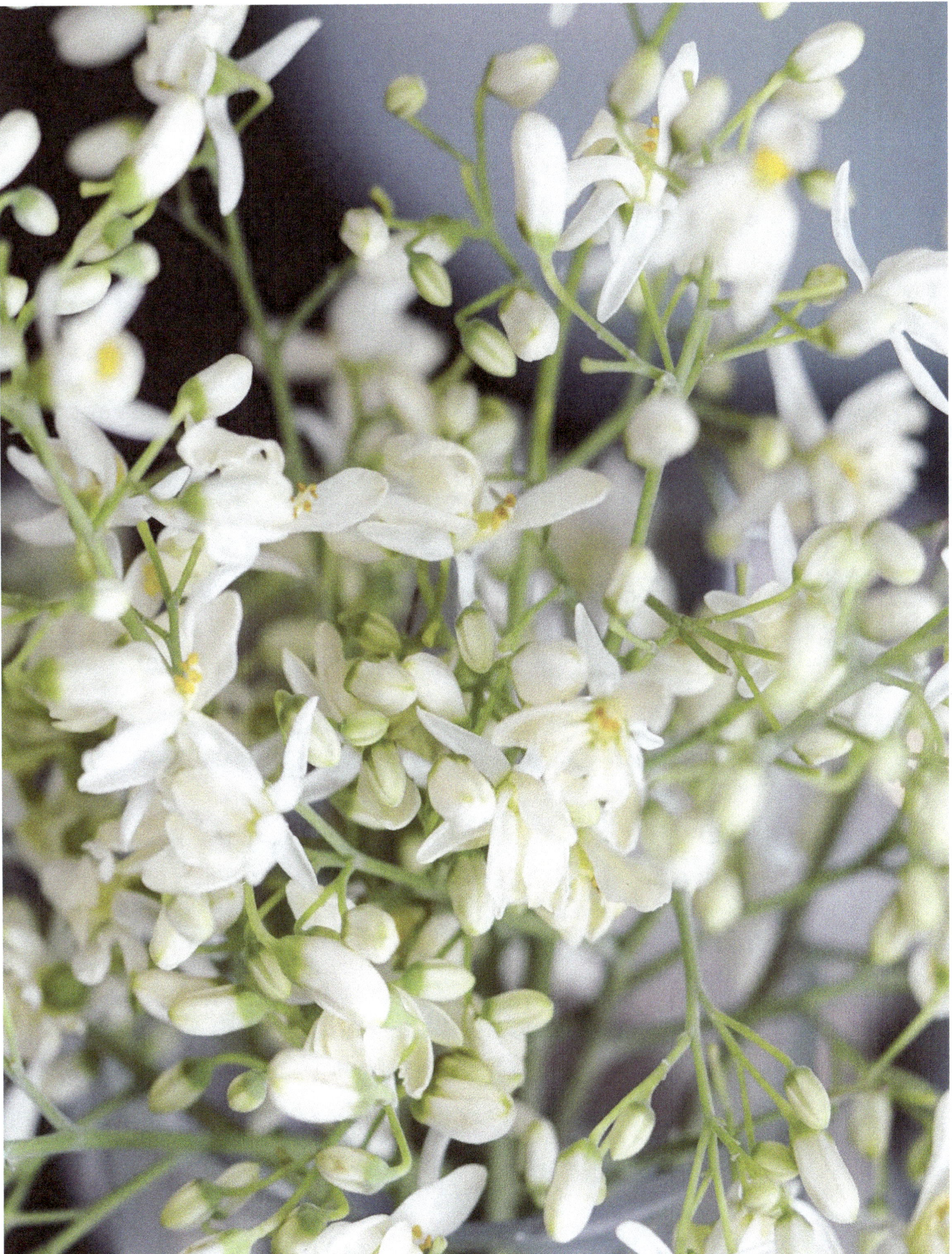

CONTENTS

RECIPES WITH MORINGA FLOWERS

RECIPES WITH MORINGA LEAVES

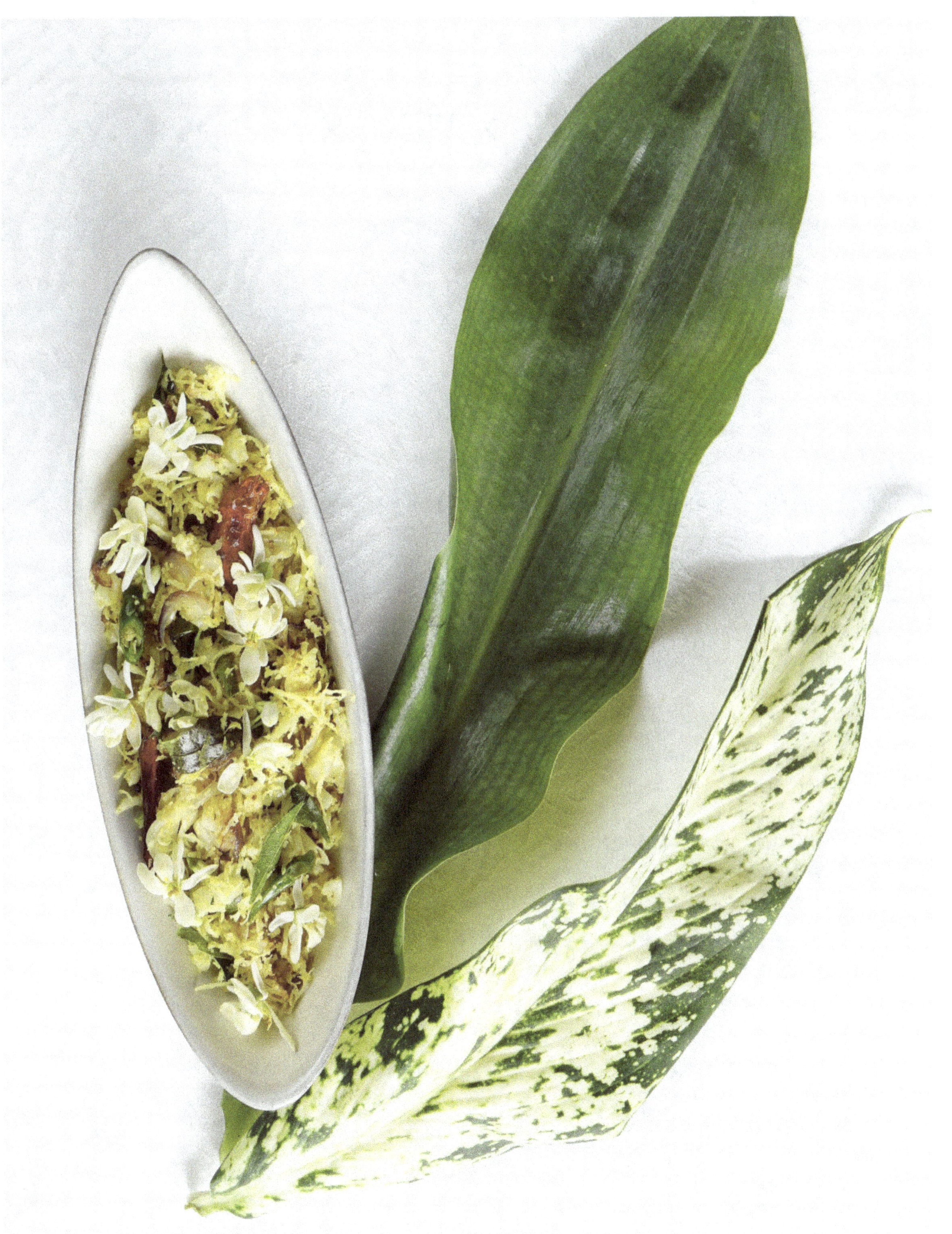

CONTENTS

RECIPES WITH MORINGA DRUMSTICKS

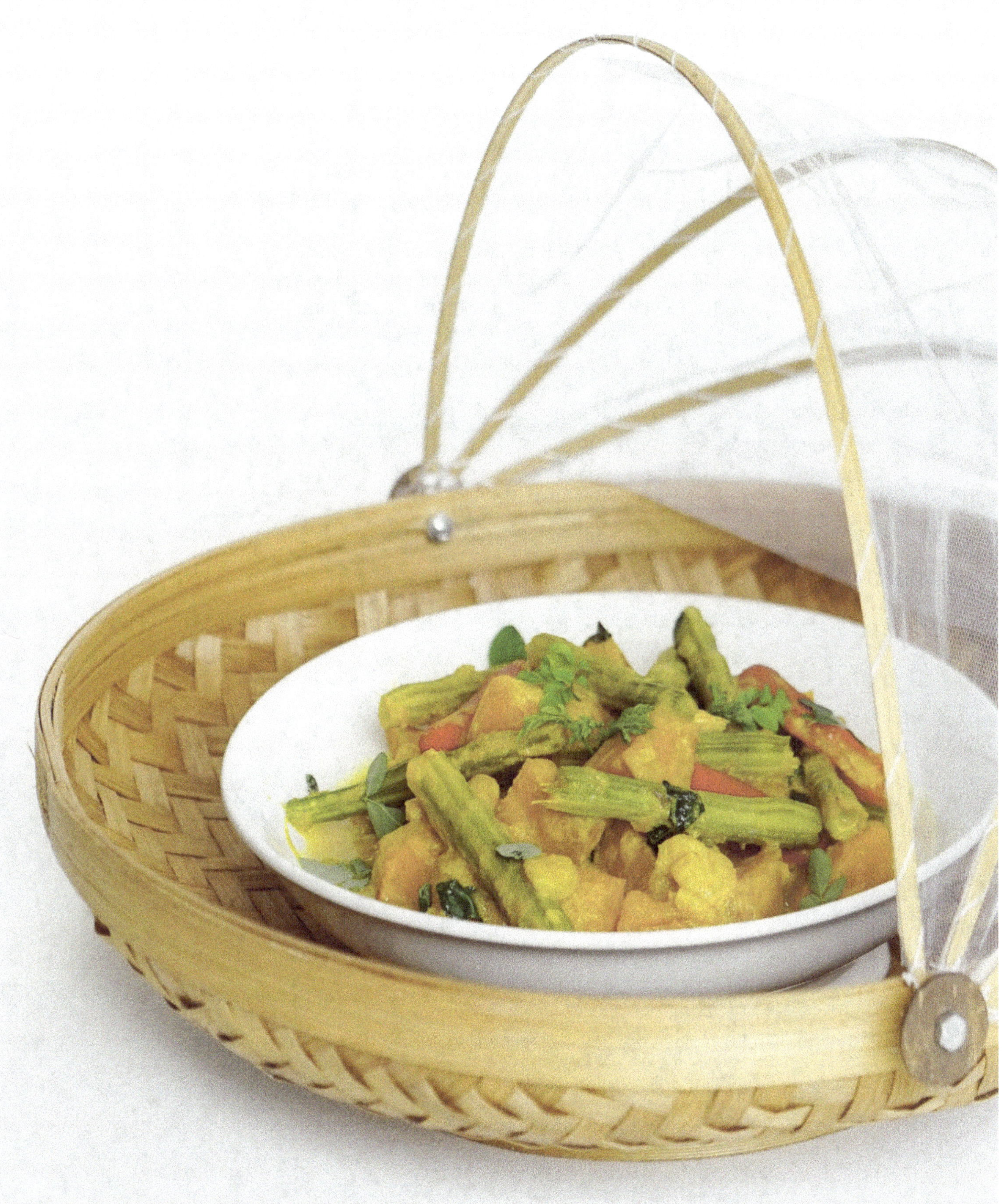

THE MIRACLE TREE

The moringa has a long and fascinating history that
spans thousands of years, and continues to be revered
for its versatility and many, many health benefits.

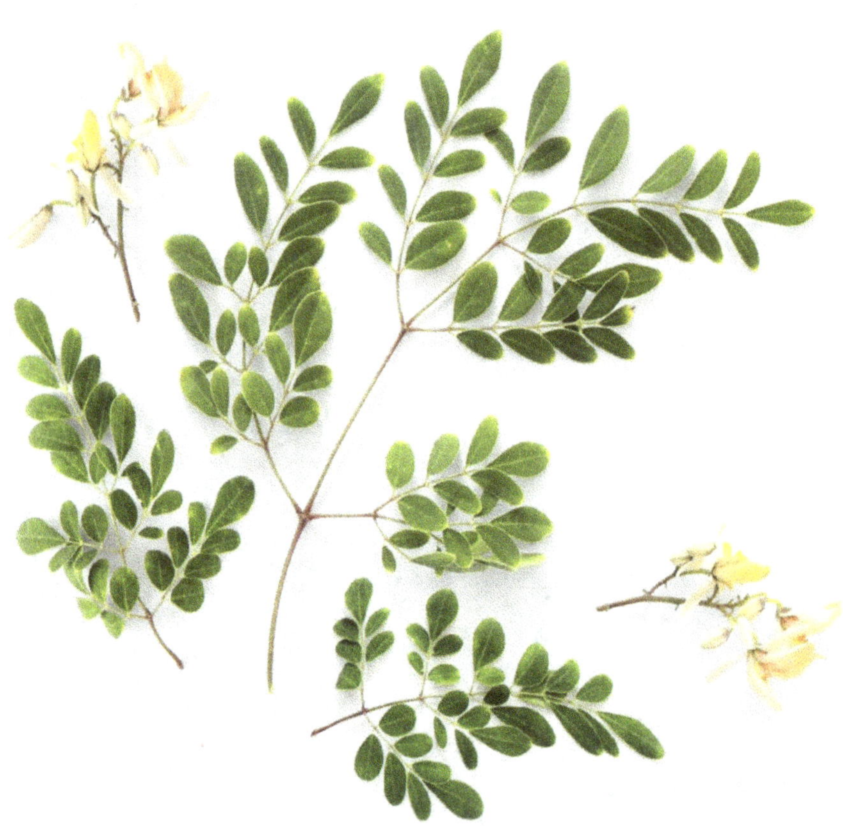

Moringa oleifera, or more commonly referred to as just moringa, also goes
by a long list of monikers—horseradish tree, drumstick tree, radish tree,
ben oil or benzolive tree, Tree of Life, arango, badumbo, caragua, sohanjna,
rawag, la mu shu, teberindo, maranga-calalu—that attest to its widespread
use and popularity around the globe. Just as long is the list of health benefits
that are attributed to it, and the fact that every part of the tree can be used
or consumed, which has led to it being widely hailed as the Miracle Tree.

"Learn character from trees, values from roots, and change from leaves"

- Tasneem Hameed

AN ANCIENT TREASURE

Native to the foothills of the Himalayas in India, the moringa tree has been cultivated and used for food and medicine for more than 4,000 years by various cultures and communities. A species of the Moringaceae family, it is a fast-growing, drought-resistant tree that can reach a height of up to 10 metres and grows in many tropical and subtropical regions around the world, including Asia, Africa, and Latin America, parts of the Caribbean, and the Pacific Islands. As it can tolerate a wide range of soil conditions, including poor and sandy soils, the moringa tree is well adapted to grow even in arid and semi-arid regions.

The moringa tree is known for its high yield and ability to thrive with minimal water, making it a valuable crop for farmers in many parts of the world. It also has merits as a sustainable and environmentally-friendly crop that can help address issues such as food insecurity and malnutrition in developing countries.

Most of all, the moringa is revered for its abundance of nutritional and medicinal properties, which have been documented in historical records and manuscripts dating back thousands of years.

In India, the ancient system of Ayurveda, which means "science of life", long recognised the healing properties of moringa and practitioners use it to promote overall health, well-being, and to treat over 300 different ailments. Most notably, Ayurvedic medicine extols the healing benefits of moringa to achieve optimal and overall wellness, including supporting the immune system, improving digestion, promoting body-mind balance, and reducing inflammation in the body.

For centuries, many in Africa have embraced the moringa as a treatment for health issues such as malaria, diabetes, and high blood pressure. At the same time, the leaves and pods of the plant are used as a food source to provide valuable nutrients to communities in areas where food is scarce. Meanwhile, in the Caribbean, moringa is a common remedy for conditions such as headaches, joint pain, and indigestion.

With growing interest and emphasis on health following the COVID-19 pandemic, this wonderfully nutrient-dense plant has been enjoying a new surge in popularity and deservedly so. Awareness of the plant's many potential health benefits has spiked in recent years and even science agrees with what moringa enthusiasts have always believed: studies have confirmed the efficacy of many traditional uses of moringa and at the same time, discovered new ways to apply different parts of the plant.

MODERN-DAY MORINGA

Today, moringa is known and loved as a superfood, and is increasingly found in health food stores, drugstores, and supermarkets in easy-to-use forms. This includes powders that can be added to food and cooking, and capsules to be taken as supplements.

Convenient as these may be to modern living and busy schedules, the best way to maximize the benefits of moringa is to consume it in its freshest, most natural form. The tree grows easily and can be cultivated in your home garden. In South-East Asia, where the tropical climate is most ideal for the moringa to thrive, it is quite common to find the tree growing in someone's backyard. If you live in colder countries, the moringa can also be grown indoors as a house plant.

The moringa tree itself is easily recognisable by its long, slender, green leaves that are slightly serrated, and its white or cream-coloured flowers. Its seeds—from which moringa oil can be extracted—are encased in long, thin pods that many fondly refer to as "drumsticks". Besides its many health and nutritional plus points, the moringa is also known as a highly versatile plant as every single part of the tree is edible and provides different types of nourishment to the human body. And here's the best part: you can very easily incorporate moringa into your life by adding it to your food, drinks, and also in self-care items like body lotions, face creams, and soaps.

Why not cultivate the moringa in your garden and harvest its parts freshly to add to your home cooking or DIY self-care remedies? In this cookbook, we will show you how you can easily incorporate this wonderful, miraculous plant into your daily life.

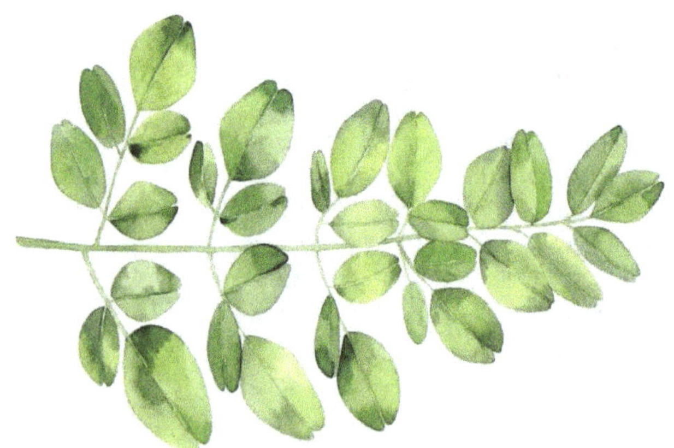

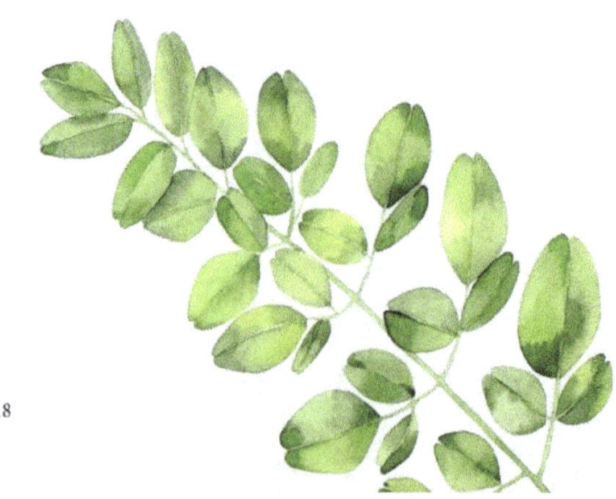

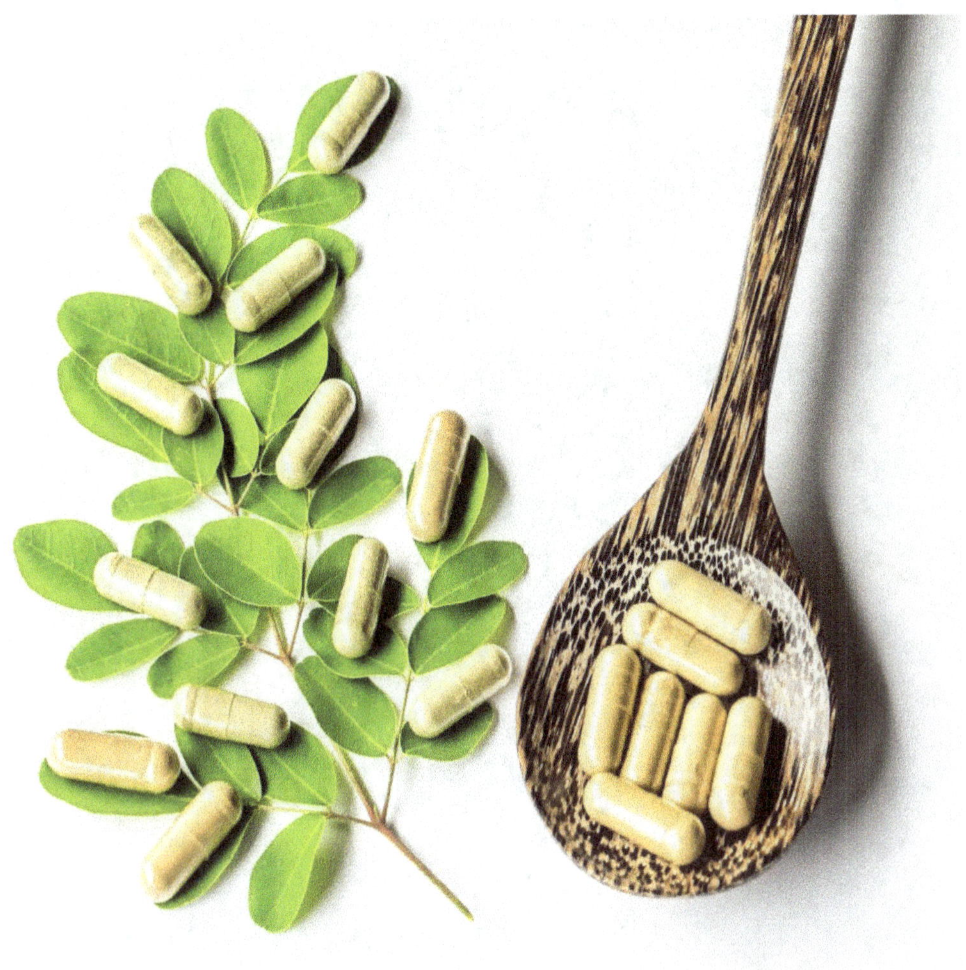

MYTHS ABOUT MORINGA

Moringa has been used for centuries in traditional medicine and has a rich cultural and historical background in many countries. Legends and myths abound about this plant and while these stories are not supported by scientific evidence, they do reflect the deep cultural significance that the moringa holds for many communities around the world.

In Indian mythology, the moringa tree is believed to have been created by the gods and is considered a sacred plant. According to the legend, the gods were searching for a cure for a deadly disease that was ravaging their people. The goddess of wealth, Lakshmi, revealed to them the healing powers of the moringa tree, which they then used to cure the disease and save their people.

In some African cultures, moringa is believed to have magical properties and is used in various rituals and ceremonies. For instance, in the Yoruba culture of Nigeria, the leaves are believed to have the power to protect against evil spirits and are often used in purification ceremonies.

Another popular belief about moringa is that it can increase a person's lifespan. This belief is believed to have originated from the fact that the plant is packed with essential vitamins and nutrients that can boost the immune system and overall health.

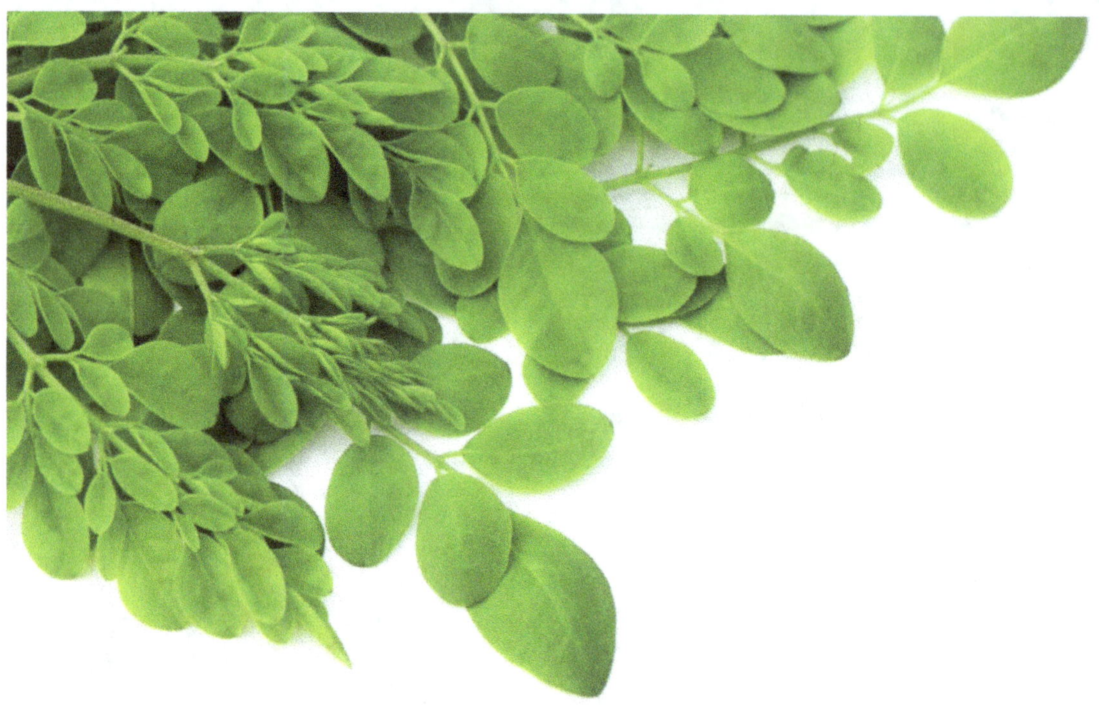

A TREE OF MANY USES

Nearly every part of the Miracle Tree is edible and usable, with each delivering different but equally nourishing benefits. Here's what you need to know to gain the most from this amazing plant.

TAKE IT, DON'T LEAF IT

Small, with oval or tear drop shapes, the leaves are the most consumed part of the tree as they are an excellent source of protein and are nutrient-dense. Slightly bitter with a grassy aroma and undertaste, they can be consumed in a variety of ways: steeped as tea, blended into smoothies, eaten raw as garnishing for soups or salads, ground into powder and added to your favourite beverages, or baked into desserts and pastries.

SO, THE SEEDS

They can be boiled and eaten as they are or like the leaves, added to soups, stews, and sauces. You can also roast the seeds for a snack and pop them as you would popcorn. Rich in antioxidants, astringent, and anti-inflammatory properties, they are known to help lower cholesterol, regulate blood sugar, fortify the immune system, and strengthen the cardiovascular system. The seeds are also used for water filtration—add them to untreated water to help separate sediment and impurities.

DRUMSTICK DELIGHT

Moringa seeds grow encased in long pods that are often known as "drumsticks" and are well loved in South Asia, where they are usually parboiled and cooked in soups, stews, stir-fries, and curries. They can also be eaten raw and said to taste similar to green beans when young, and like asparagus when the pods are older.

TRACE THE ROOTS

The roots are considered the most nutrient-rich part of the tree and have been consumed therapeutically as far back as early Roman, Greek, and Egyptian times. They can be grated and served as a condiment that tastes like horseradish. As the roots contain high levels of fibre, protein, vitamins, and minerals, they are often prescribed as a remedy for malnutrition. However, caution must be exercised if eating a large amount due to the presence of spirochin, which can lead to paralysis.

FLOWERLICIOUS!

Delicate, with tiny white petals, moringa flowers grow in small clusters. They are considered a delicacy and loved for their mushroom-like taste. When steeped as a tea, they are considered a cure for the common cold while according to Ayurveda, the flowers can be made into a pressed juice to treat urinary tract infections and improve lactation for breastfeeding.

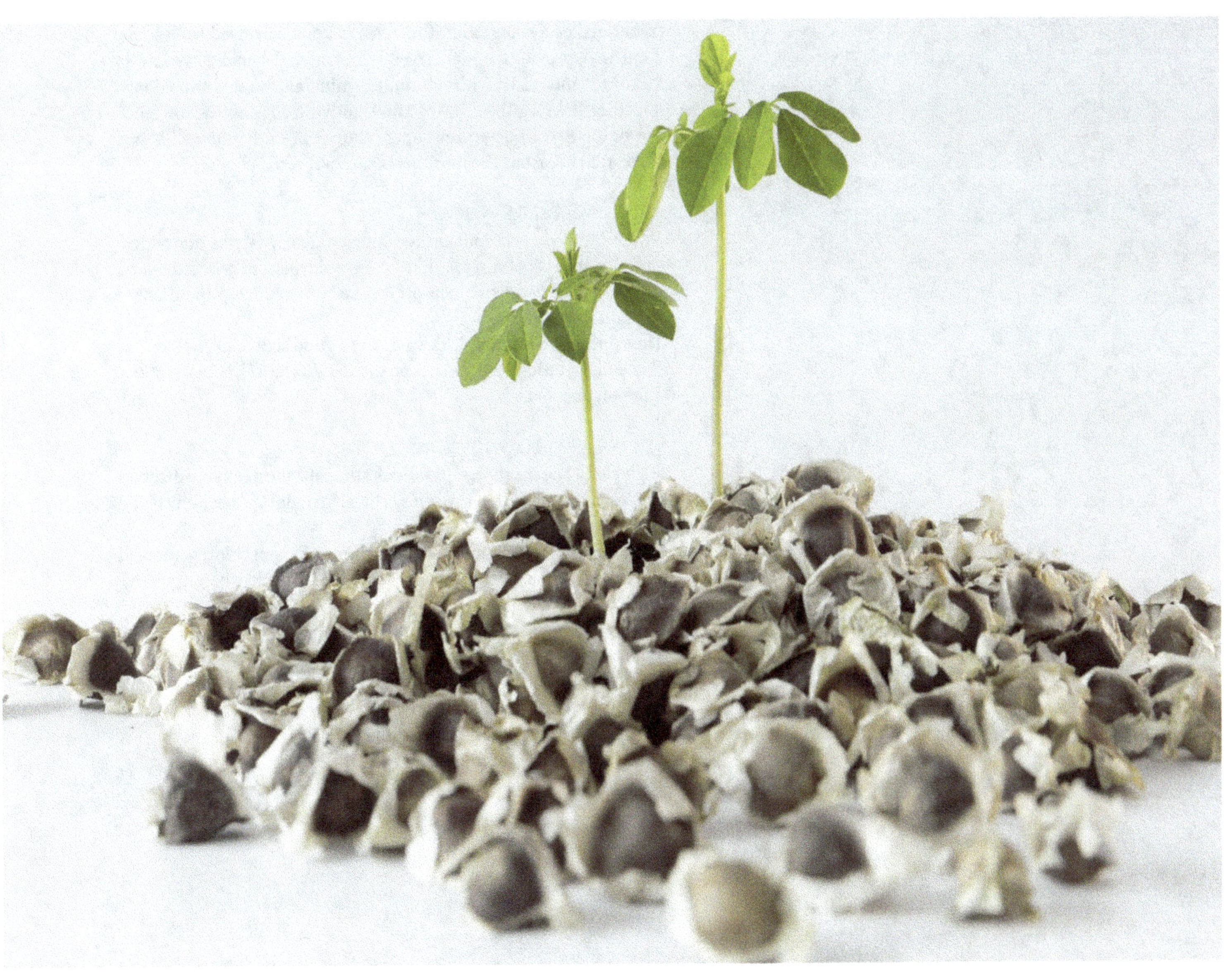

11 REASONS MORINGA IS CONSIDERED A SUPERFOOD

They call it the Miracle Tree or
Tree of Life, and this is why.

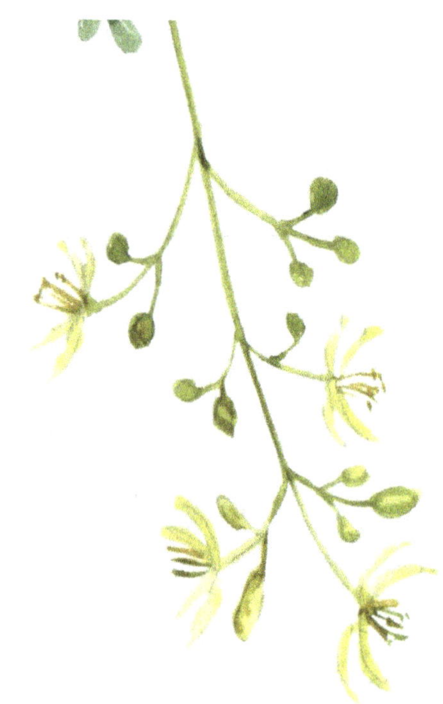

What makes a superfood? This term is popularly used to describe food that provides a high level of nutritional benefits, is low in calories, and rich with vitamins, minerals, and antioxidants. Moringa ticks all these boxes and rightly belongs on the esteemed list of foods considered the super heroes of health and well-being. Here are 11 reasons the moringa is such a revered plant:

#1 FIGHTS FREE RADICALS

When the body accumulates too much oxidative stress due to free radicals, the risk of diseases like heart problems and type 2 diabetes increases. Antioxidants help protect cells by reducing the damage brought on by free radicals.

How does moringa help? Its leaves are a good source of compounds that deliver antioxidative benefits, such as Vitamin C, beta-carotene, and polyphenols.

#2 LOWERS BLOOD SUGAR LEVELS

High blood sugar can lead to serious ailments, most notably diabetes and heart diseases. That's why it's critical to maintain a healthy blood sugar level at all times.

How does moringa help? Thanks to the presence of chlorogenic acid and isothiocyanates, the moringa plant helps regulate blood sugar.

#3 REDUCES INFLAMMATION

Inflammation is important to help the body heal from infection and injury, but if it's sustained over a long period, one becomes susceptible to all kinds of chronic illnesses including cancer.

How does moringa help? The isothiocyanates found in moringa is believed to have anti-inflammatory qualities.

#4 LOWERS CHOLESTEROL

To keep your heart healthy, it is important to regulate cholesterol and moringa has been found to be beneficial for this.

How does moringa help? It contains hypocholesterolemic, which helps lower lipid, and antiatherescotic that prevents plaque build-up in artery walls.

#5 IMPROVES LIBIDO

Low or reduced sex drive can be caused by a multitude of factors, including stress, anxiety, and depression.

How does moringa help? Reduce stress, increase blood flow, boost testosterone, enhance moods—moringa is believed to have these properties that contribute towards improving one's sexual health and desires. Additionally, it is a great source of potassium and antioxidants, which makes it a potential aphrodisiac.

#6 BOOSTS ENERGY

If you want a caffeine-free energy booster, moringa could be the answer to your prayers.

How does moringa help? The cocktail of vitamins (B, C, and D) along with iron found in moringa encourage better energy production and sustain long-term energy while optimizing metabolic health.

#7 FEEDS THE BRAIN

Having trouble remembering things or focusing on work or tasks? Maybe it's not due to lack of motivation but nutrient deficiency in the brain.

How does moringa help? Moringa is considered great brain fuel due to its amino acid and vitamin profile, which includes tryptophan that is said to help improve cognitive functions like learning and remembering things.

#8 FIGHTS THE CLOCK

Wouldn't you love to be able to keep premature wrinkles at bay and maintain youthful-looking skin? Some believe that the moringa is an elixir of youth!

How does moringa help? Moringa contains a high amount of flavonoids and polyphenols, and both are known to have anti-ageing properties.

#9 REGULATES BLOOD PRESSURE

Hypertension is a common malady, especially among the older population due to years of unhealthy lifestyle choices, lack of regular exercise, or as the result of health issues like diabetes or obesity.

How does moringa help? Moringa contains quercetin, which has anti-hypertensive qualities that helps stabilise blood pressure. Taken alongside a nutritious diet and with regular exercise, moringa is can be helpful to those with high blood pressure.

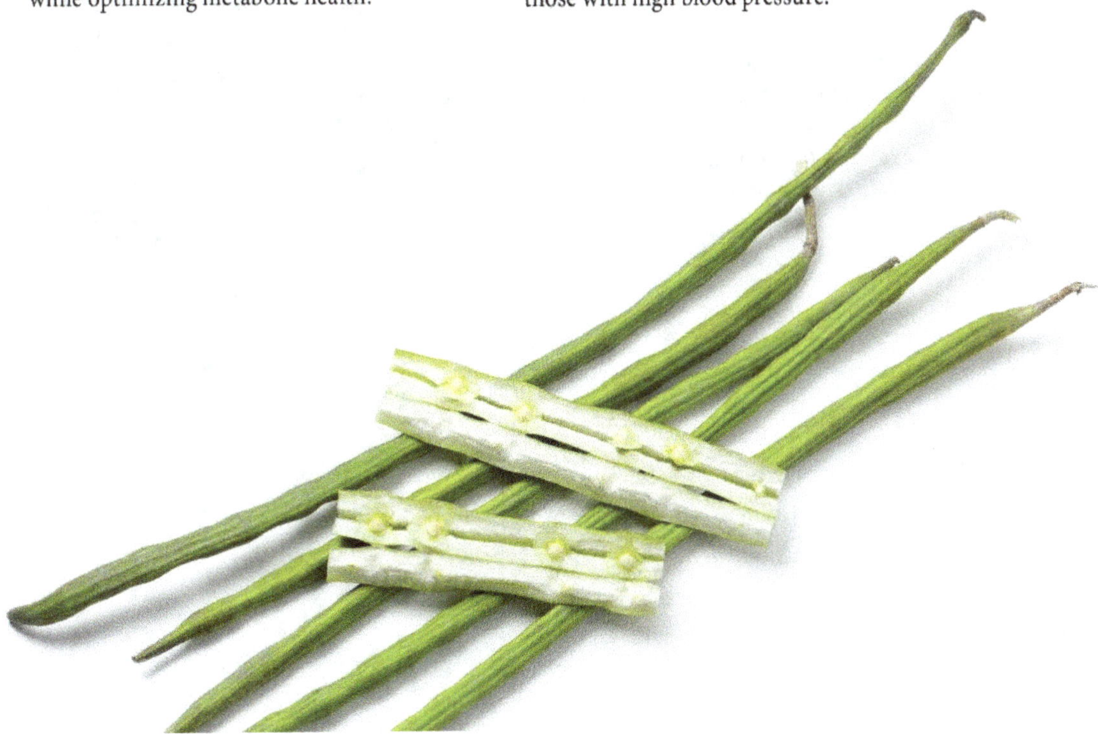

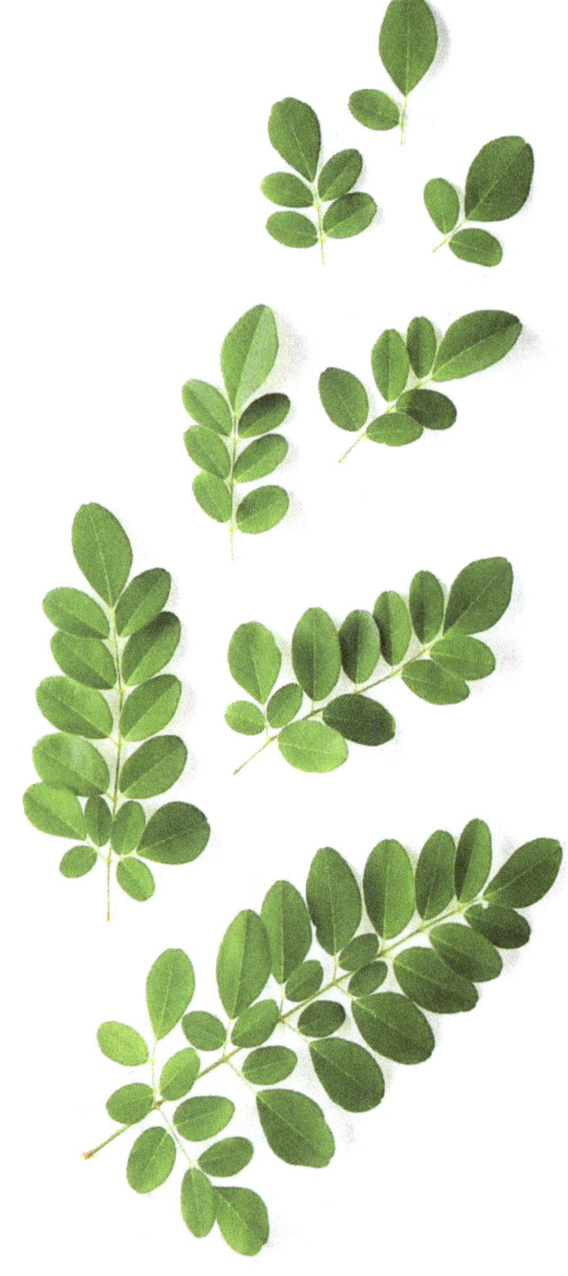

#10 PROMOTES BETTER GUT HEALTH AND DIGESTION

If constipation or irregular bowel movement is causing you distress, you can look into adding more soluble fibre in your diet to optimize your gut microbiome.

Soluble fibre not only keeps you fuller for longer but also eases constipation.

How does moringa help? Rich in both soluble and insoluble fibres, moringa helps create a conducive environment in your gut for beneficial bacteria to grow and help move things along.

#11 PROTECTS THE LIVER

The liver is the body's main detox channel. It is therefore crucial to ensure that your liver is functioning well and protected from oxidative stress or damage.

How does moringa help? Moringa is rich in polyphenols, which can give the liver a much-needed boost.

MORINGA IN NUMBERS

90+
Contains more than 90 types of nutrients

>40
Rich in over 40 antioxidants

300+
Helps treat more than 300 diseases and illnesses

IS MORINGA SAFE FOR EVERYONE?

• The leaves and seed pods are generally safe but do practise general caution if you are not used to consuming moringa and consult your doctor beforehand
• If consumed in large quantities, some eaters may experience stomach upset and other digestive issues
• Women who are pregnant or nursing should avoid consuming the root, bark, and flowers
• Moringa may interact with some medications, so check with your physician before adding it to your diet

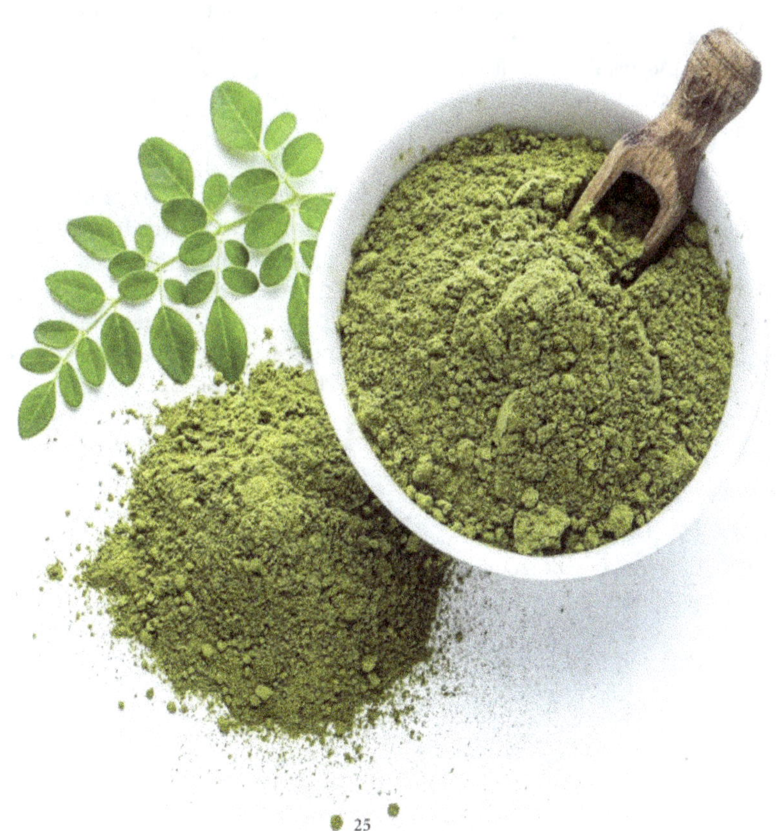

THE BEST MEDICINE, DISPENSED BY NATURE'S PHARMACY

Moringa's abundance of medicinal properties and health benefits
is legendary. Rich in vitamins, minerals, and antioxidants,
it's an excellent remedy for a variety of ailments.
Plant a moringa tree in your garden and it would be akin to
having a ready source of multi-vitamin at your doorstep!

DIABETES

Moringa leaves contain compounds that help increase insulin secretion and improve glucose tolerance, thereby regulating blood sugar levels and helping to manage diabetes.

Usage Consume the leaves in fresh or dried form. The latter includes moringa powder, which you can add to any food or drink you consume. Moringa oil can also be used topically on the skin to treat diabetic wounds and ulcers.

INFLAMMATION

With its anti-inflammatory properties, moringa is an effective natural remedy for conditions such as arthritis, gout, and other conditions that cause swelling.

Usage Grind moringa leaves into a paste and apply it topically to inflamed areas. Moringa oil can be massaged into the skin to reduce joint pain and inflammation.

ANAEMIA

Moringa is a rich source of iron, which is essential for the formation of red blood cells. Regular consumption of moringa can help prevent anemia.

Usage Consume moringa leaves and pods raw, cooked, or in the form of powder or supplements.

RESPIRATORY PROBLEMS

Due to the plant's anti-inflammatory properties, which can help reduce inflammation in the lungs and airways, moringa has been used to treat a range of respiratory problems: asthma, bronchitis, and other lung-related conditions.

Usage Sip on moringa tea (add ginger, honey, or lemon for added benefits) or apply moringa oil onto the chest and throat.

CHOLESTEROL

Moringa leaves contain compounds that help lower LDL (bad) cholesterol levels and promote the production of HDL (good) cholesterol.

Usage Drink moringa tea or add moringa powder to your food or drink to reduce cholesterol levels.

DIGESTIVE PROBLEMS

The leaves and pods are rich in fibre, which helps improve digestion and prevent constipation, to alleviate digestive problems such as constipation, bloating, and diarrhoea.

Usage Consume moringa leaves and pods raw or cooked, or in the form of powder or supplements.

EYE PROBLEMS

Moringa contains high levels of Vitamin A, which is essential for maintaining healthy eyesight. Regular consumption can help with eye problems such as cataracts and macular degeneration.

Usage Consume the leaves raw or cooked, or in the form of powder or supplements to help improve eye health.

HIGH BLOOD PRESSURE

Its ability to relax blood vessels and promote better blood flow make moringa an effective remedy to reduce high blood pressure.

Usage Brew the leaves into a tea and consume it daily, or add moringa powder to your food and drinks. Moringa seeds are known to have the same effects on blood pressure.

SKIN PROBLEMS

Moringa has been found to be effective in treating skin problems such as acne, eczema, and psoriasis thanks to the plant's anti-inflammatory and antibacterial properties.

Usage Moringa oil can be used topically to treat skin problems such as acne, eczema, and psoriasis. Apply moringa oil directly to the affected areas and massage gently.

CANCER

The plant's leaves and seeds contain compounds that can help prevent the growth and spread of cancer cells.

Usage Consume moringa leaves and seeds raw or cooked, or in the form of powder or supplements to help fight cancer.

Whether you're looking to improve your health or simply add more nutrients to your diet, moringa can be a fantastic remedy—do consult with your doctor before using it to treat any health issue, especially if you're taking medication or have underlying health conditions.

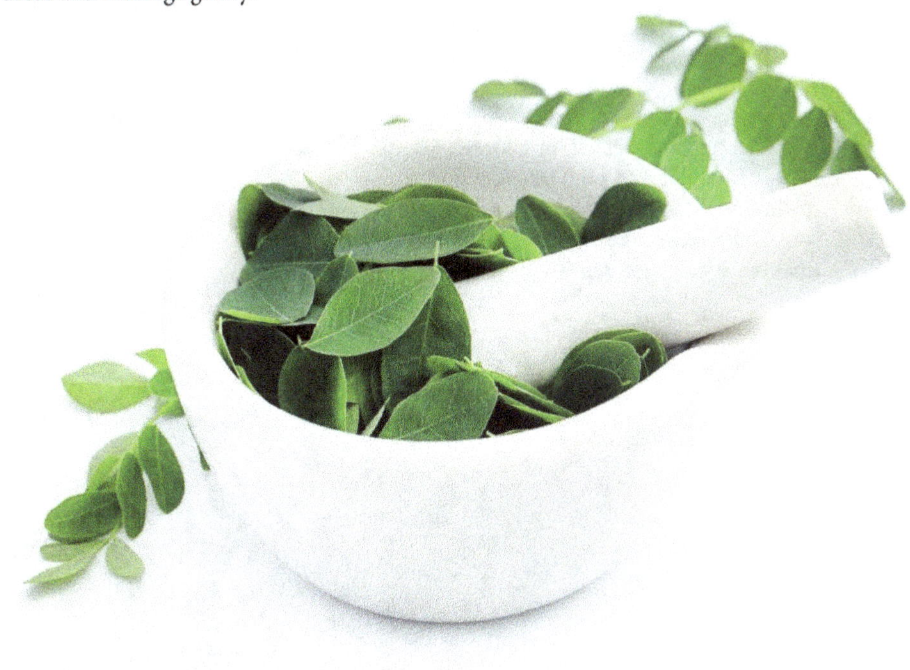

FEED YOUR SKIN, MAKE IT GLOW

Moringa's powerful cocktail of vitamins, antioxidants, and other skin-loving nutrients makes it a fantastic ingredient for skincare products: from cleansers to moisturisers, face masks to serums.

Moringa's healing properties lend themselves well to nurturing and nourishing the skin, both on the inside and outside. Antioxidants found in the plant can help shield the skin from damage caused by free radicals and environmental stressors, keeping the signs of ageing at bay. You will be blessed with plump, radiant, and youthful skin that radiates a glowing complexion.

Moringa is also a natural cleanser and can be used to remove impurities and excess oil from the skin. Use it as an exfoliator (scrub gently!) to remove dead skin cells and reveal brighter, smoother skin.

Another notable benefit of moringa is its ability to soothe and calm irritated skin. The plant has anti-inflammatory properties that can help to reduce redness and inflammation, making it ideal for sensitive or acne-prone skin.

Moringa can also be used in its pure oil form for the face and body. Due to its rich moisturising effects and high oleic acid content, moringa oil is excellent for keeping the skin hydrated and moisturised.

Enriched with brightening properties thanks to high levels of Vitamin C, moringa can help reduce the appearance of dark spots and hyperpigmentation, leading to a brighter, more even skin tone.

TOP TIP

When choosing skincare products that contain moringa, do a patch test before applying onto the entire face or body.

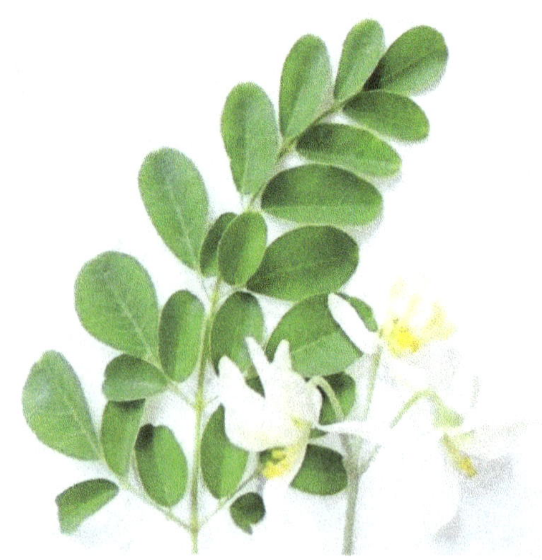

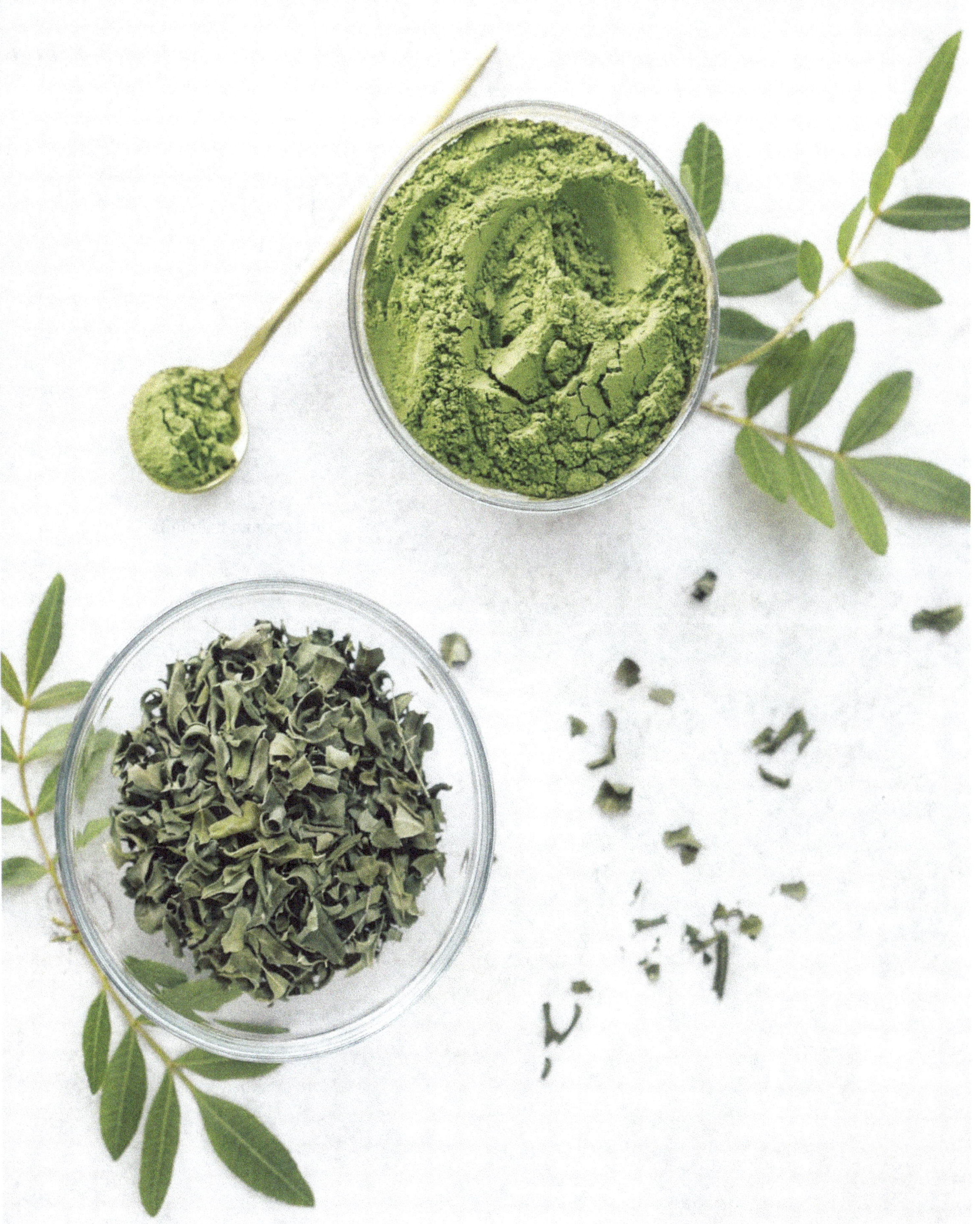

TINY LEAVES WITH HUGE BENEFITS

Take a look at how moringa stacks up against other
food in terms of key nutrients and vitamins.

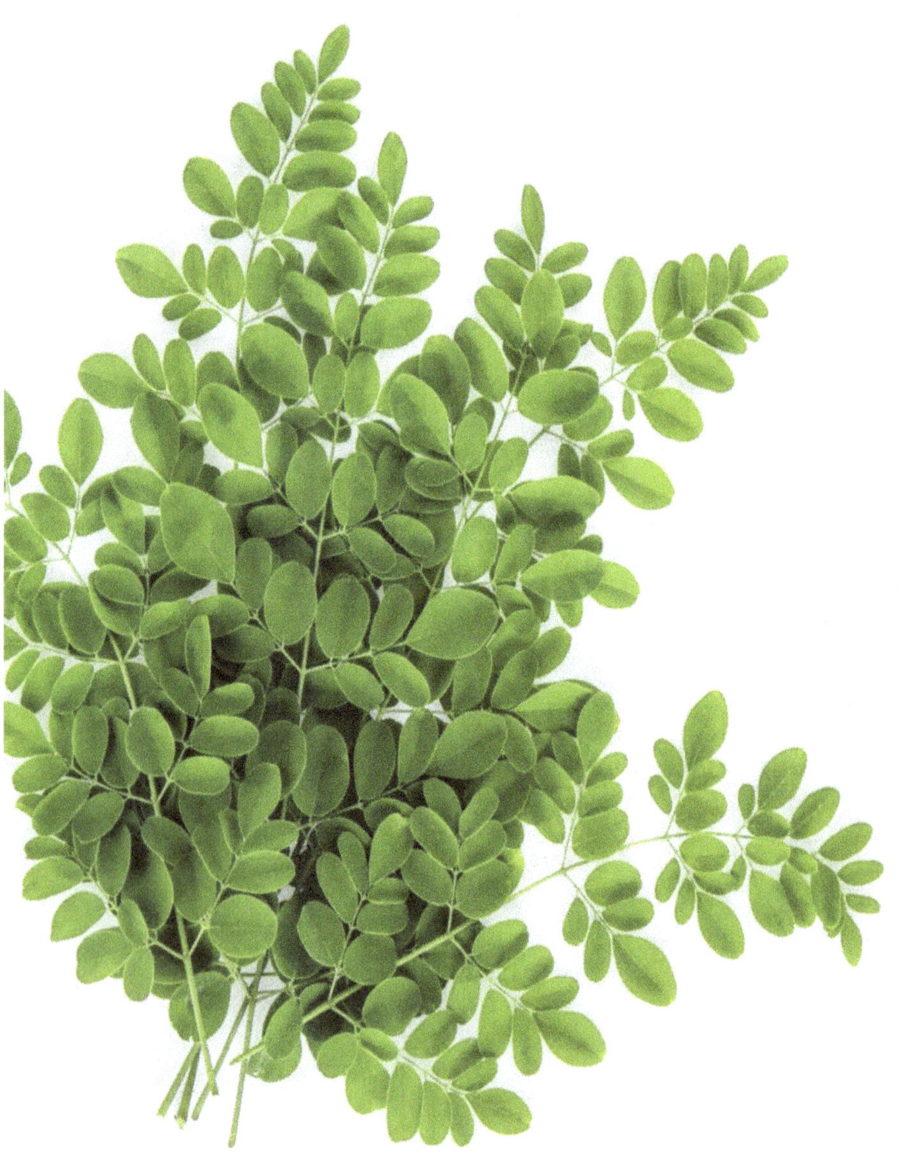

17X
More calcium than milk

10X
More Vitamin A than
carrots

7X
More Vitamin C than
oranges

15X
More potassium than
bananas

9X
More protein than yogurt

25X
More iron than spinach

Moringa leaves—they can be consumed fresh, dried, or in powder form—are packed with amino acids that enable the body to build protein. Fresh leaves have up to 75% moisture content that, when dried, is significantly reduced while the nutrients become more concentrated. Moringa leaves crushed into powder form is an extremely high protein-rich option.

In fact, just 10g of moringa powder will provide:

2.5g protein
0.6g fat
2.6g carbohydrates
2.4g fibre
198mg calcium
49.5mg magnesium
4.5mg iron
2.3g Vitamin C

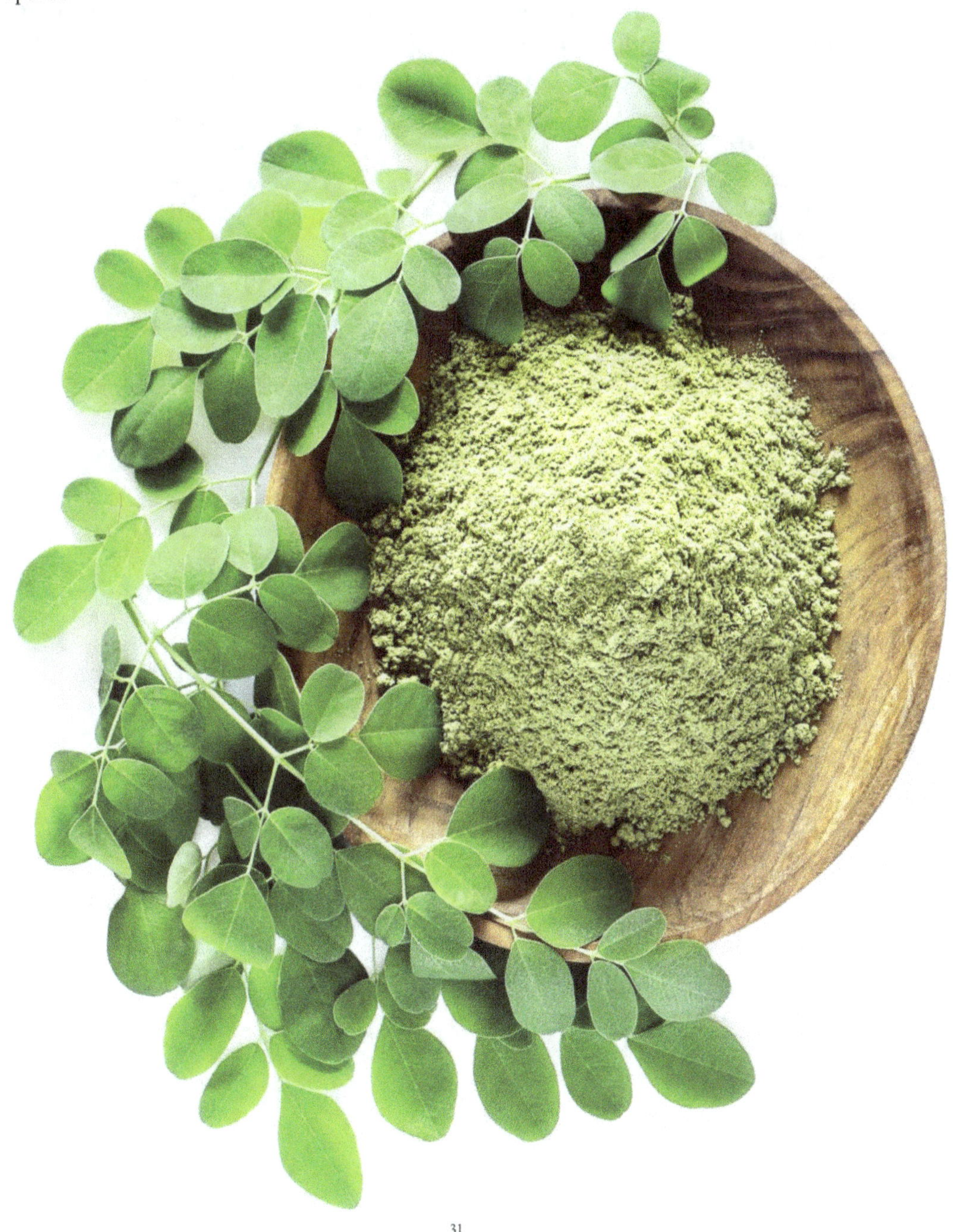

BIG BENEFITS FOR YOUR LITTLE ONES: MORINGA FOR CHILDREN

In the pursuit of raising healthy and resilient children, the role of proper nutrition cannot be overstated. Among the treasure trove of nature's offerings, *Moringa oleifera* emerges as a powerhouse of essential nutrients, a potential ally in ensuring the well-being and development of your little ones. Here are some ways moringa benefits children:

PROTECTS THEIR IMMUNITY

Packed with vital vitamins, minerals, and proteins, moringa can contribute significantly to your young ones' overall growth and immune system support. The abundance of Vitamin A enhances vision, while the rich Vitamin C content fortifies children's immunity, safeguarding them from common infections.

IMPROVES GENERAL WELL-BEING

Moringa's immune-boosting properties are especially vital for children, whose developing immune systems need robust support. Essential nutrients like iron and zinc contribute to the production of immune cells, while antioxidants help combat oxidative stress and inflammation, promoting overall wellness.

BETTER BONE HEALTH AND GROWTH

The high calcium and phosphorus content in moringa plays a pivotal role in bone development and density, which is a critical aspect of children's growth. These minerals, coupled with exceptional protein content, provide the foundation for strong bones and muscles, ensuring that children reach their optimal physical potential.

BOOSTS COGNITIVE POWERS

Children's cognitive development is a key concern for parents and caregivers. Moringa's rich antioxidant content, including Vitamin E, supports brain health and function. Its neuroprotective properties aid in maintaining cognitive clarity and focus, contributing to enhanced learning and academic performance.

ENHANCES DIGESTIVE HEALTH

Moringa's role in promoting a healthy digestive system is equally noteworthy. Its fibre-rich leaves and pods aid in maintaining regular bowel movements and preventing constipation. The tree's natural antimicrobial properties help ward off digestive ailments, ensuring children's comfort and well-being.

BALANCES BLOOD SUGAR

The prevalence of childhood obesity and diabetes is a growing concern. Moringa has been studied for its potential to regulate blood sugar levels, making it a valuable addition to a balanced diet aimed at preventing these metabolic disorders in children.

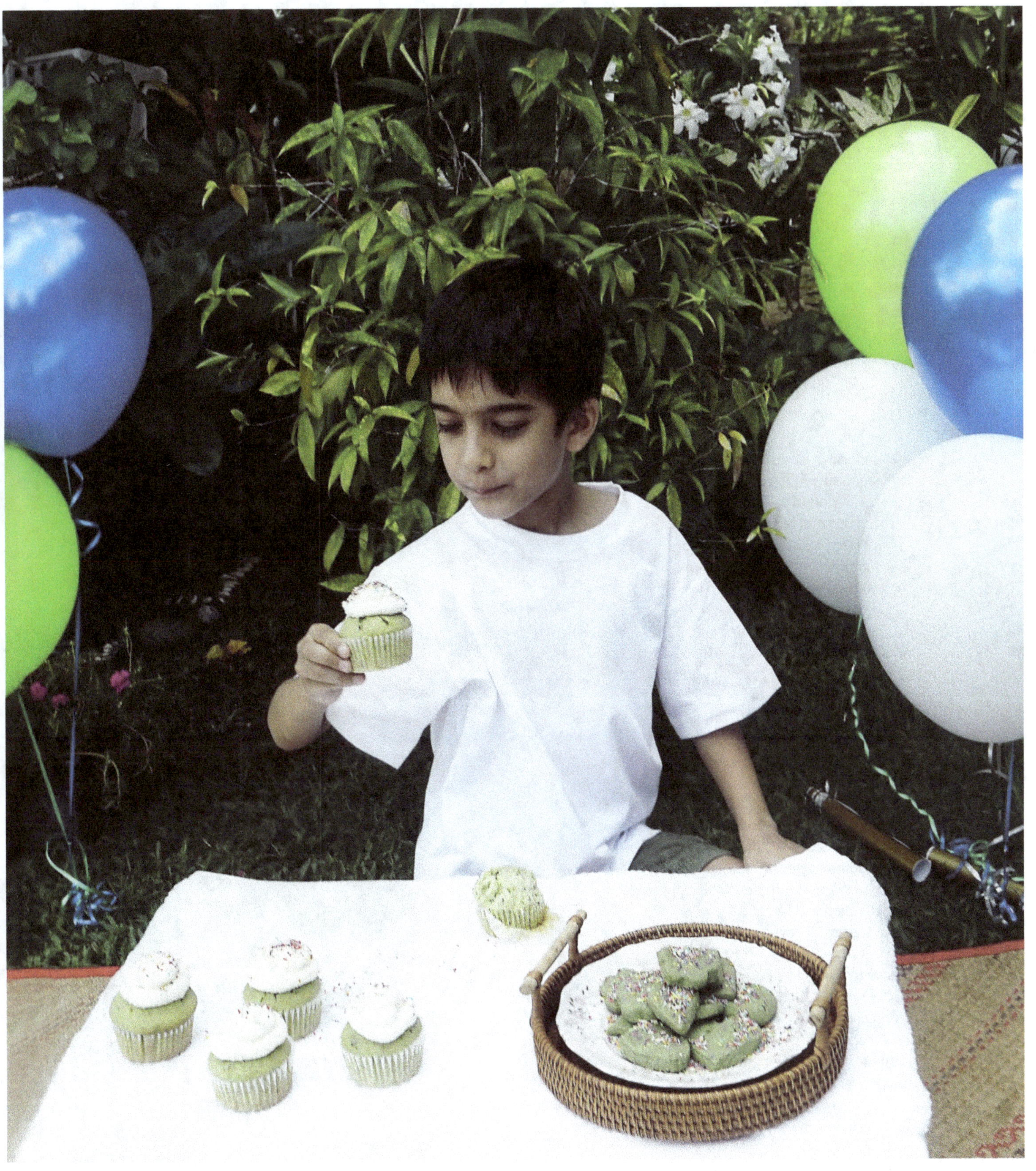

"To eat is a necessity, but to eat intelligently is an art"
- La Rochefoucald

5 CLEVER WAYS TO GET YOUR KIDS TO ENJOY MORINGA

1. Blend moringa leaves into vibrant fruit smoothies for an instant nutrient boost. The vibrant colors and sweet flavors of berries, bananas, and a splash of juice (see pg 124 for recipe) ensure that your little ones will gulp down all the goodness without a second thought.

2. Turn moringa into refreshing and visually-appealing popsicles. Mix moringa powder with coconut water or yogurt, add a touch of honey for sweetness, pour into popsicle molds, and freeze. Your kids will relish these delightful treats while reaping the benefits of this superfood.

3. Sneak some moringa goodness (in the form of powder or blended leaves) into their favourite desserts—like cupcakes or muffins. Your little ones will happily dig into them and be none the wiser about the healthy twist!

4. Simply toss cooked chickpeas with a hint of olive oil and a sprinkle of moringa powder, then roast until crispy. This crunchy delight is a great way to introduce moringa into their snacking routine.

5. Transform breakfast into a nutrient-packed adventure with Moringa Pancakes (see pg 80 for recipe) for an extra dose of vitamins. Top with their favorite fruits and a drizzle of honey to make mornings a delight.

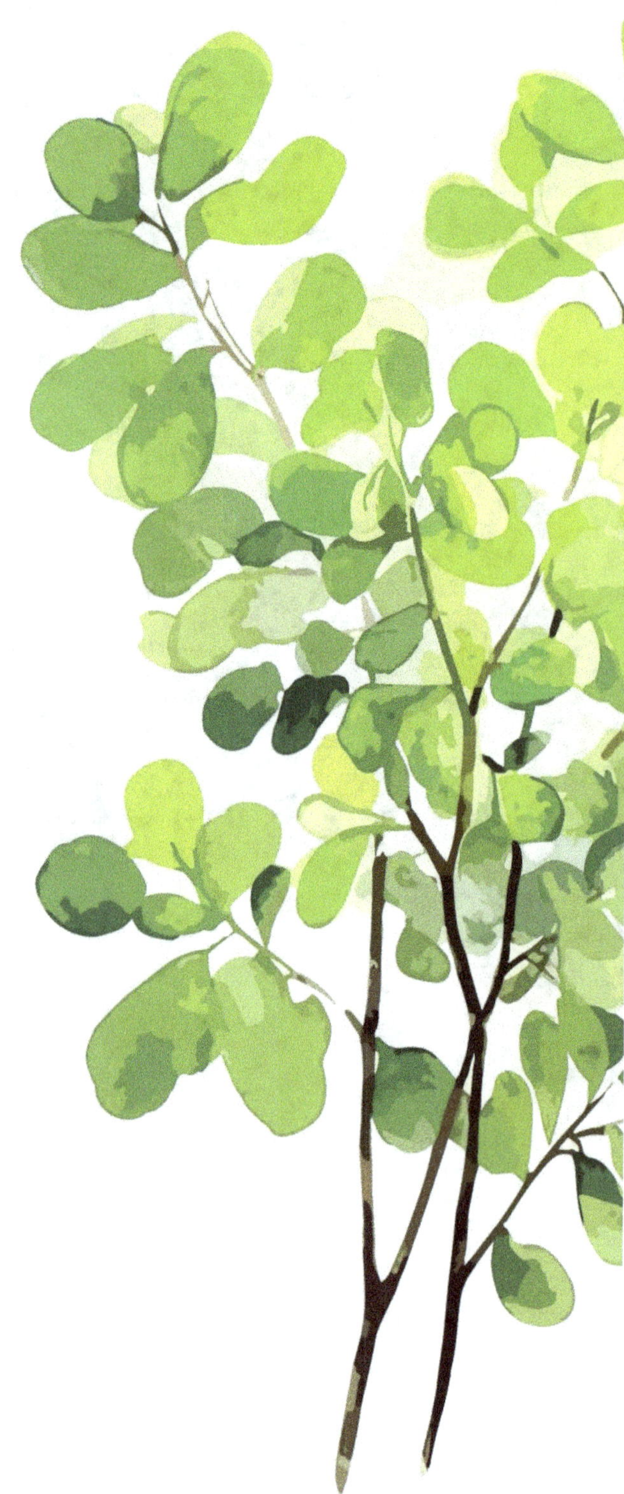

PAW-SITIVE HEALTH: MORINGA FOR PETS

As a pet owner, you care for your furry companions' health and well-being as much as your own so why not let them enjoy the wholesome goodness of moringa too? It's safe for most domestic animals like cats and dogs and can be easily incorporated into their diets to elevate their vitality.

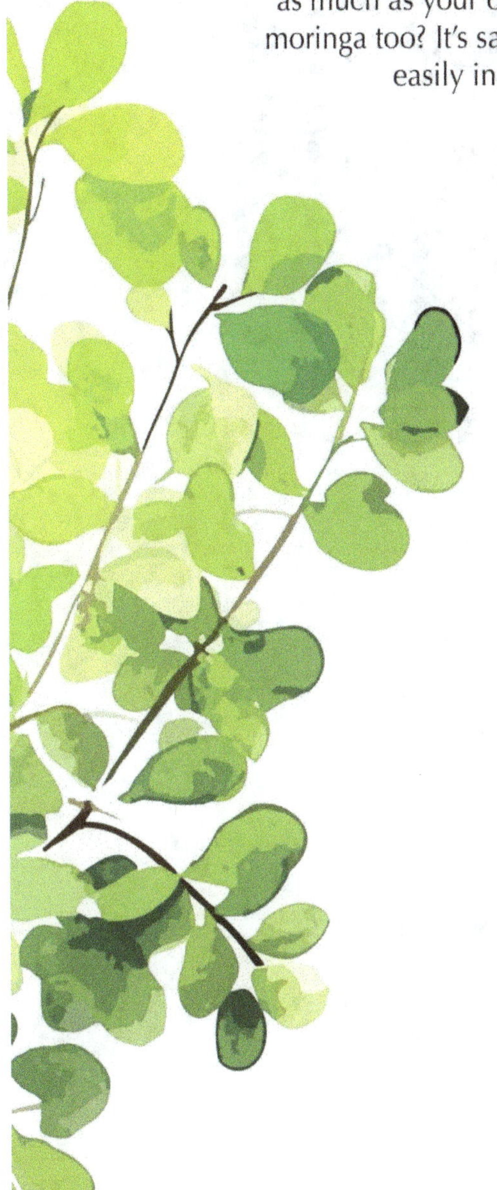

Here's how moringa benefits your beloved pets:

BOOSTS IMMUNITY, FIGHTS INFECTIONS

Moringa's array of vitamins, minerals, antioxidants, and essential nutrients—including vitamins A, C, and E—as well as minerals like calcium and iron can contribute to a pet's overall health. It bolsters their immune system and safeguards them against common infections, keeping them sprightly and active.

IMPROVES JOINT HEALTH AND MOBILITY

For ageing pets or those prone to joint issues, moringa's anti-inflammatory properties can offer relief and improved mobility. Its natural compounds help alleviate discomfort, making it an attractive option for pets experiencing joint stiffness or arthritis.

PROMOTES DIGESTIVE HARMONY

Just as in humans, moringa can aid in promoting digestive wellness for pets. The fibre-rich leaves can support regular bowel movements and alleviate digestive disturbances, ensuring that your pets enjoy optimal comfort.

SHINY COATS AND HEALTHY SKIN

Moringa's high content of protein and amino acids can help foster lustrous coats and healthy skin, adding an extra touch of radiance to your pets' appearance.

REGULATES WEIGHT AND ENERGY LEVELS

Moringa's role in metabolism regulation may assist in maintaining a healthy weight for pets, which is crucial for their overall well-being. Its ability to provide sustained energy can also be beneficial, ensuring that your pets remain active and engaged.

Note: Consult a veterinarian before introducing any new supplements into your pet's diet

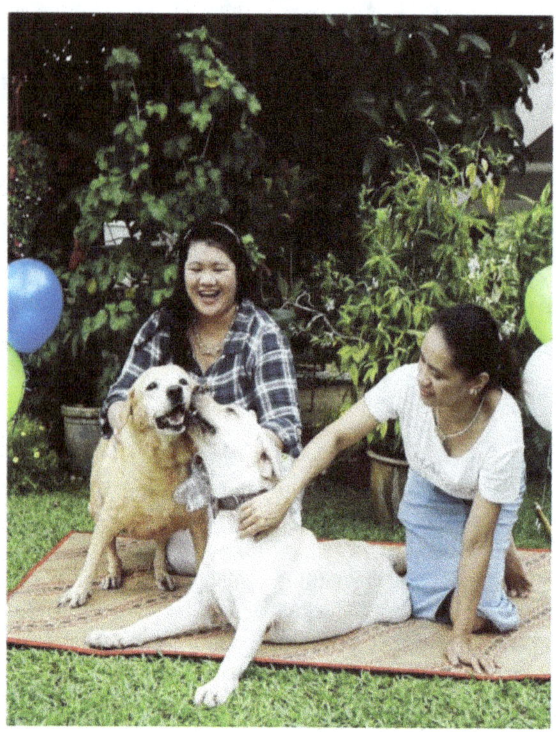 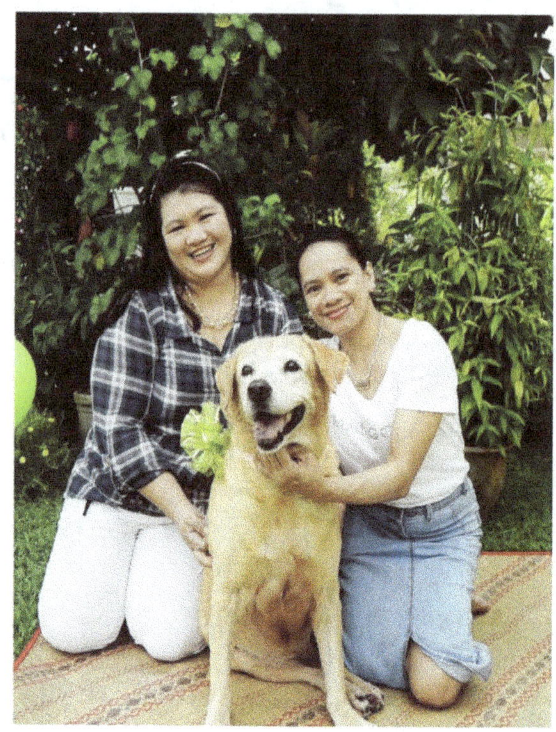

1. Sprinkle a small amount of moringa powder over your pet's regular food. Start with a tiny pinch and gradually increase the amount as they become accustomed to the taste. This simple addition can introduce a host of essential nutrients into their diet.

2. Mix moringa powder with pet-friendly ingredients like peanut butter, oats, and pumpkin puree. Shape into bite-sized treats and bake for a nutritious reward.

3. Simmer moringa leaves or powder in water, then strain to create a flavorful broth. Pour over their kibble or freeze into ice cubes for a refreshing treat on hot days.

4. Blend moringa powder or leaves with pet-safe fruits like banana, blueberries, and yogurt. Serve as a smoothie or pour into silicone molds for frozen smoothie bites that are as tasty as they are nutritious.

5. Create a mixture of cooked lean meat, steamed vegetables, and a sprinkle of moringa powder or leaves. Mix this concoction into their food to provide an extra dose of vitamins and minerals.

Remember, every pet is unique, so start with small amounts of moringa and monitor their response. With these simple yet inventive approaches, you can enhance your pet's nutrition and contribute to their vibrant well-being with the power of moringa.

Note: Do consult with a veterinarian before introducing any new supplements to your pet's diet

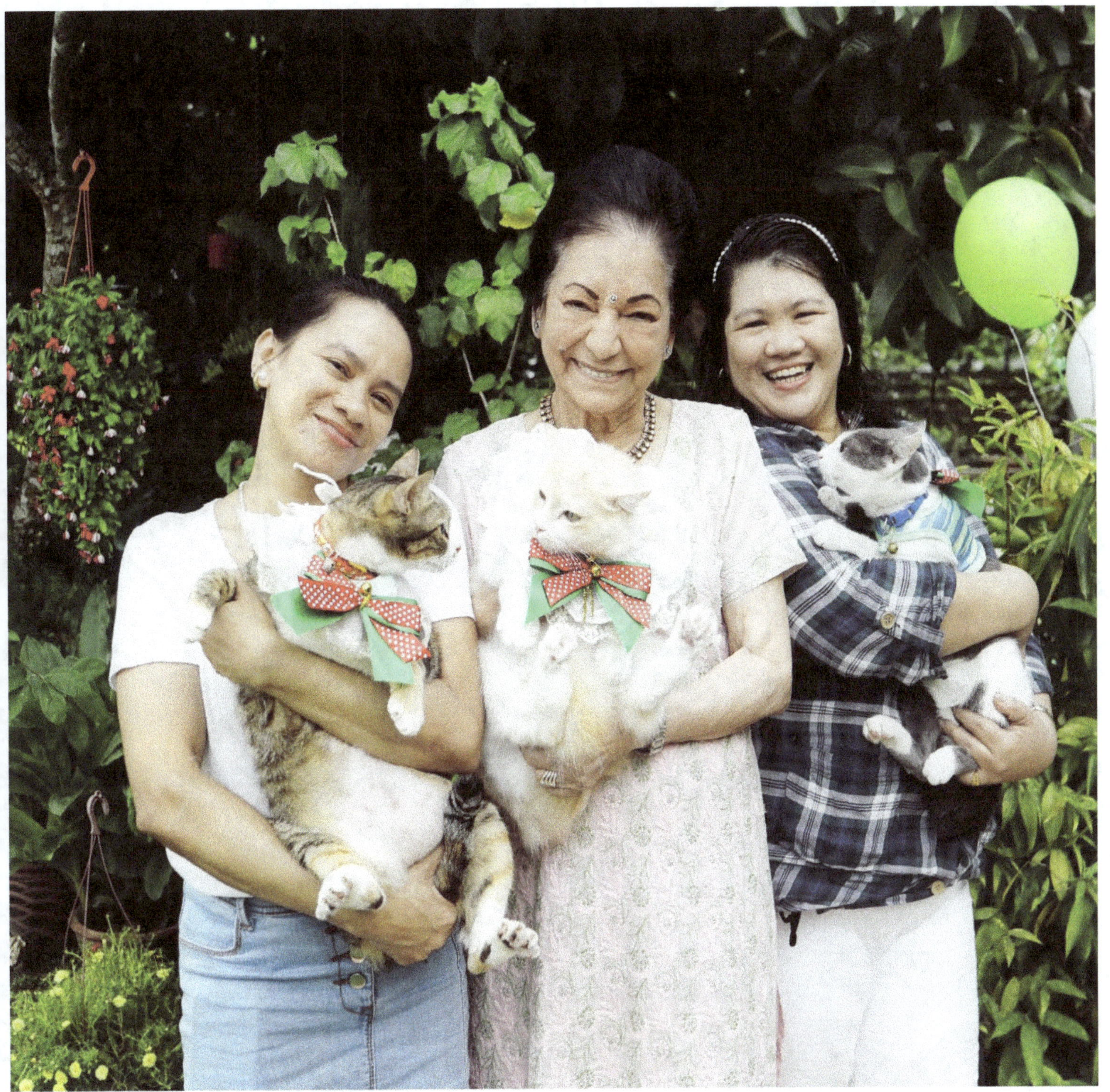

Mohana, flanked by her helpers Christine (left) and Lyn (right) and their beloved kitties

"Pets are humanising. They remind us we have an obligation and responsibility to preserve and nurture and care for all life"
- James Cromwell

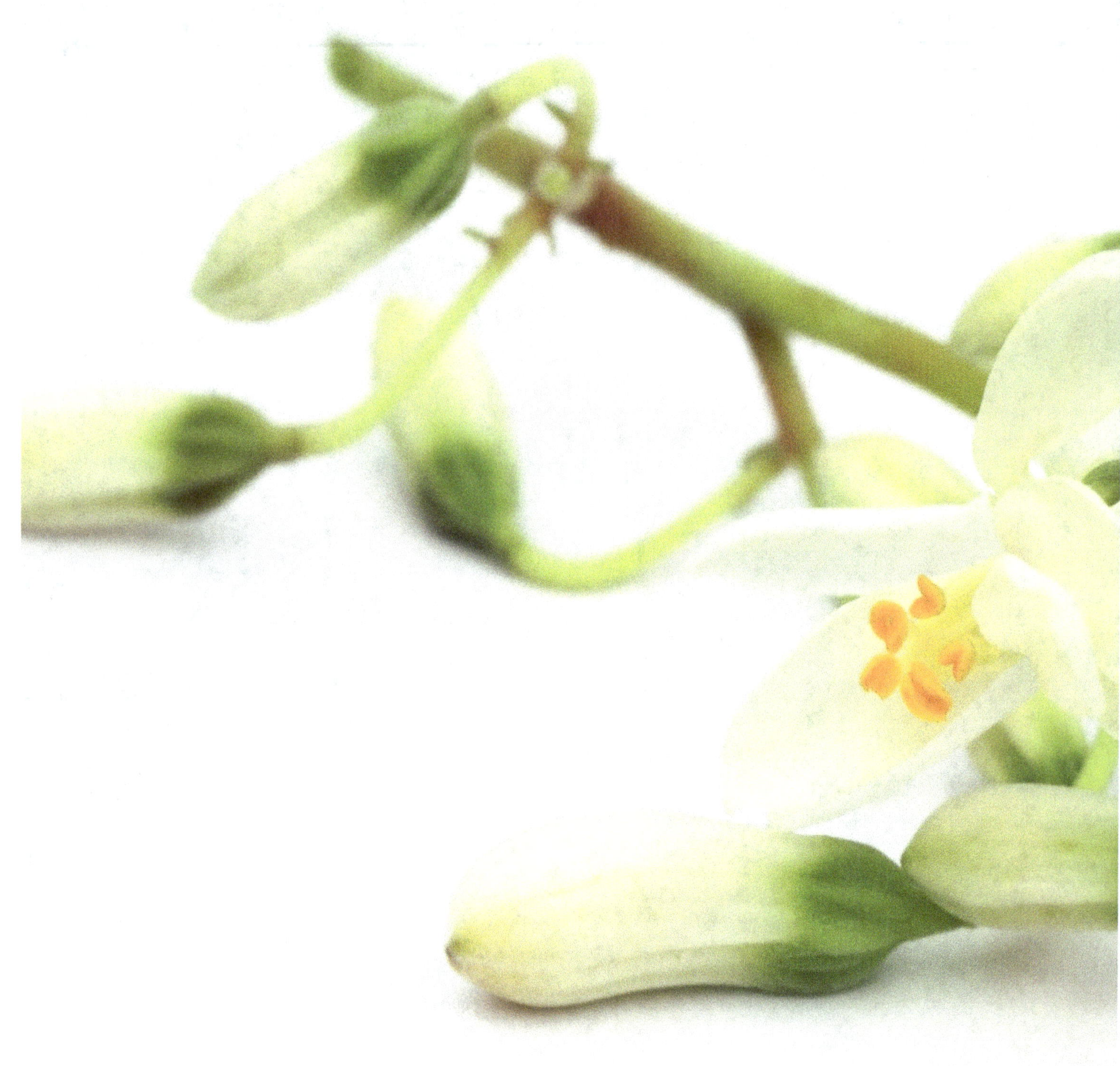

MORINGA FLOWERS

5 THINGS TO KNOW ABOUT MORINGA FLOWERS

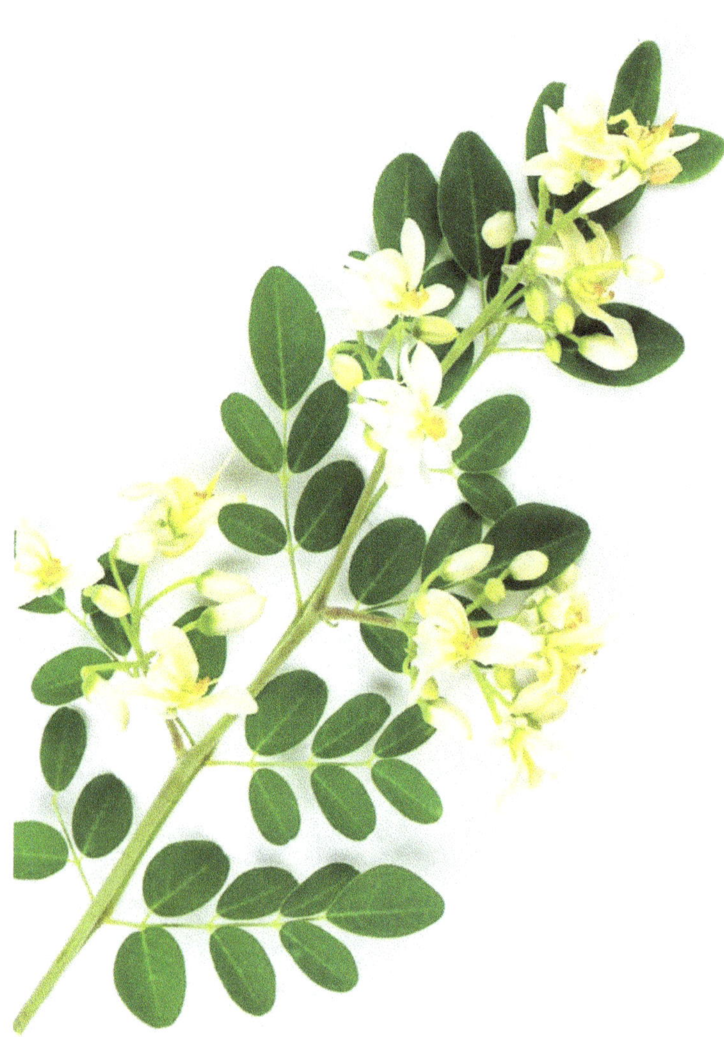

Moringa flowers are small, averaging two centimeters in diameter, and are found hanging in delicate clusters from the branches of the moringa tree. Each flower contains five soft, thin, and white petals—sometimes flushed with yellow—growing in multiple directions. The petals also surround slender stamens with bright yellow pollen attached to the anthers.

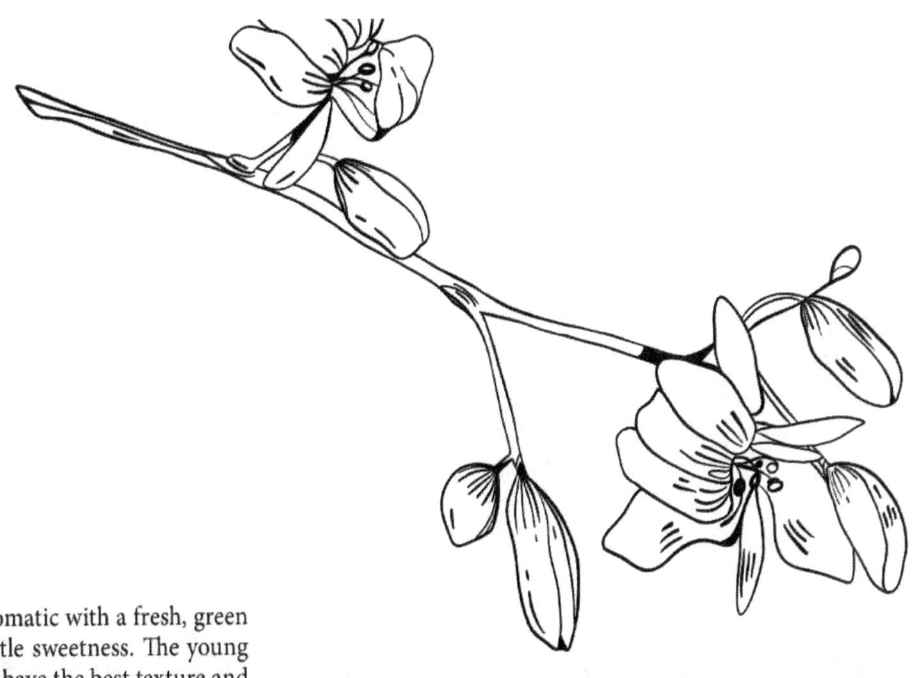

#1

Young flowers are aromatic with a fresh, green scent and have a subtle sweetness. The young flowers are known to have the best texture and taste. When cooked, they develop a flavour that is like a combination of asparagus and mushrooms. They have a soft, delicate texture and a taste profile that's quite distinctly their own—tender, mild, succulent, and juicy.

#2

Moringa flowers can be added to any of your favourite dishes, especially to replace mushrooms. They are also perfect for adding to stir-fries. Make sure to thoroughly clean them before cooking by soaking them for at least 10 minutes. Add the flowers only during the last few minutes of cooking. Keep tossing and mixing the ingredients so that the flowers won't burn.

#3

Moringa flowers should be used immediately after harvesting for the best quality and flavour; they can keep for a couple of days when stored in an airtight container in the refrigerator. In cooking, add them at the last minute as overcooking will compromise their nutritional qualities.

#4

You can also dry the flowers and store them in an airtight container. This way, they can keep for up to one year.

#5

Moringa flowers are also considered a delicacy in the Pacific Islands. In Haiti, they are often used as a remedy for colds.

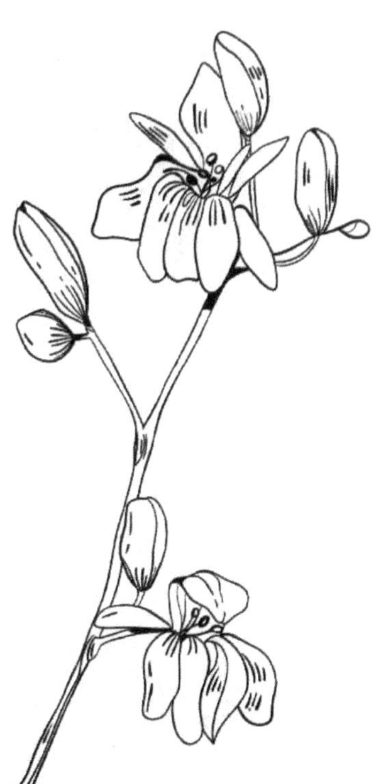

Moringa Flower Pickle

Tangy, crispy, and full of umami, this amazing pickle really opens up one's appetite. Have it as a snack on its own or serve it as an accompaniment for a meal with rice.

Ingredients
(Fills up a 500 ml glass jar)
200gm moringa flowers
200gm lotus stem, thinly sliced
1 large bulb of garlic, peeled and halved lengthwise
6-8 large chilli peppers (less hot variety), cut into bite-sized slices
⅓ cup mustard oil
3 tbsp apple cider vinegar
2 tbsp turmeric powder
3 tbsp mustard powder
1 tbsp fenugreek powder
1 tsp nigella seeds, crushed lightly
1 tsp *ajwain* (carom) seeds, crushed lightly
1-2 tbsp red chilli powder
3 tbsp salt

Method
1. Boil 1 litre of water in a deep pan with 1 tsp of salt.
2. Dip the sliced lotus stem in the boiling water for a couple of minutes and strain. Set aside.
3. Dip the drumstick flowers into the boiling water for a few seconds. Set aside.
4. Mix all ingredients in a large bowl.
5. Transfer into a sterilized glass jar.
6. Top with more mustard oil if the ingredients don't settle down and a thin layer of oil floats on top.
7. Cover the jar with a thin muslin cloth and the jar lid.
8. Place jar in a cool place away from direct sunlight.
9. After 24 hours, the pickle is ready to be served.

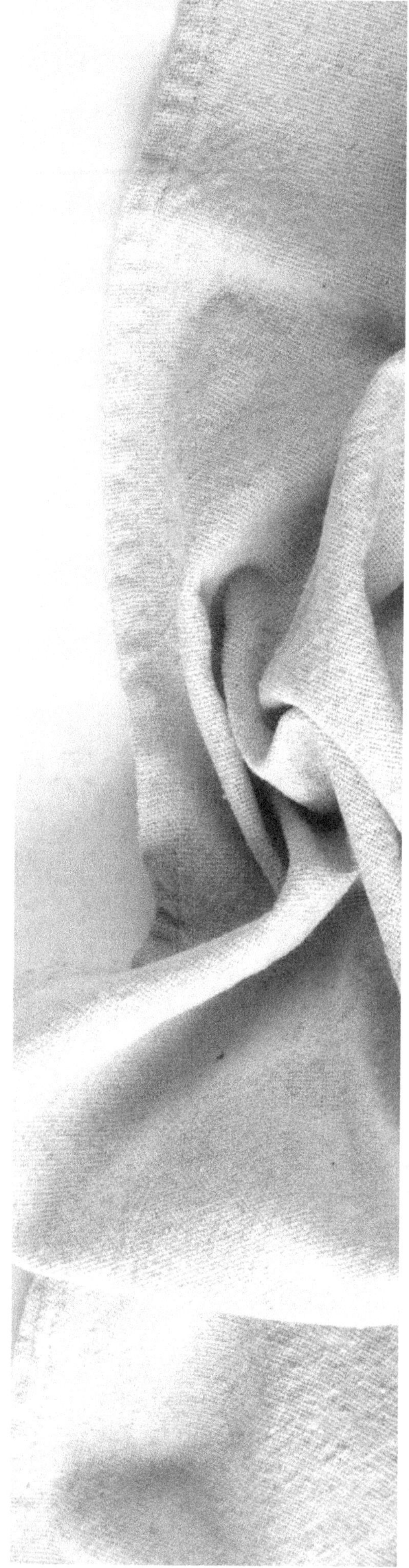

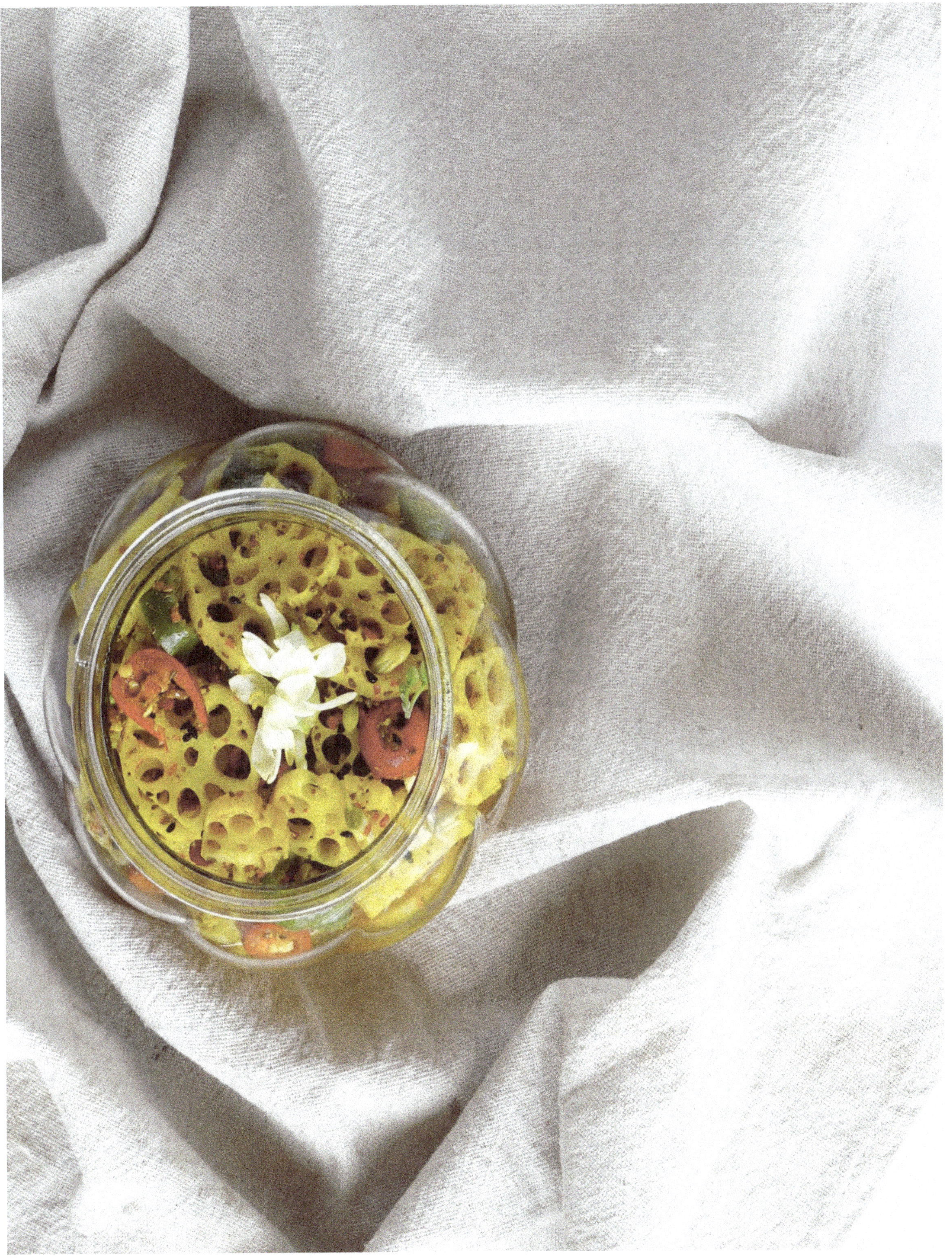

Moringa Flower Thoran

Thoran is the heart of Kerala cuisine, a stir-fried dish that traditionally features cabbage and coconut but you can prepare it using any vegetable or edible flower.

Ingredients
1 cup moringa flowers
5 shallots
1 green chili
1 stalk curry leaves
1 tsp oil
½ tsp mustard seed
1 dried red chilli
½ tsp turmeric powder
2 tbsp freshly grated coconut

Method
1. Heat oil in a heavy pan.
2. Add mustard seeds.
3. When they start popping, add the dried chilli, curry leaves, onions, green chilli, and turmeric powder.
4. Cook till the onions turn colour.
5. Toss in the moringa flowers.
6. Mix well and add salt to taste.
7. Cover and cook for about 5-10 minutes.
8. Stir in 2 tbsp grated coconut.
9. Cook for a minute.

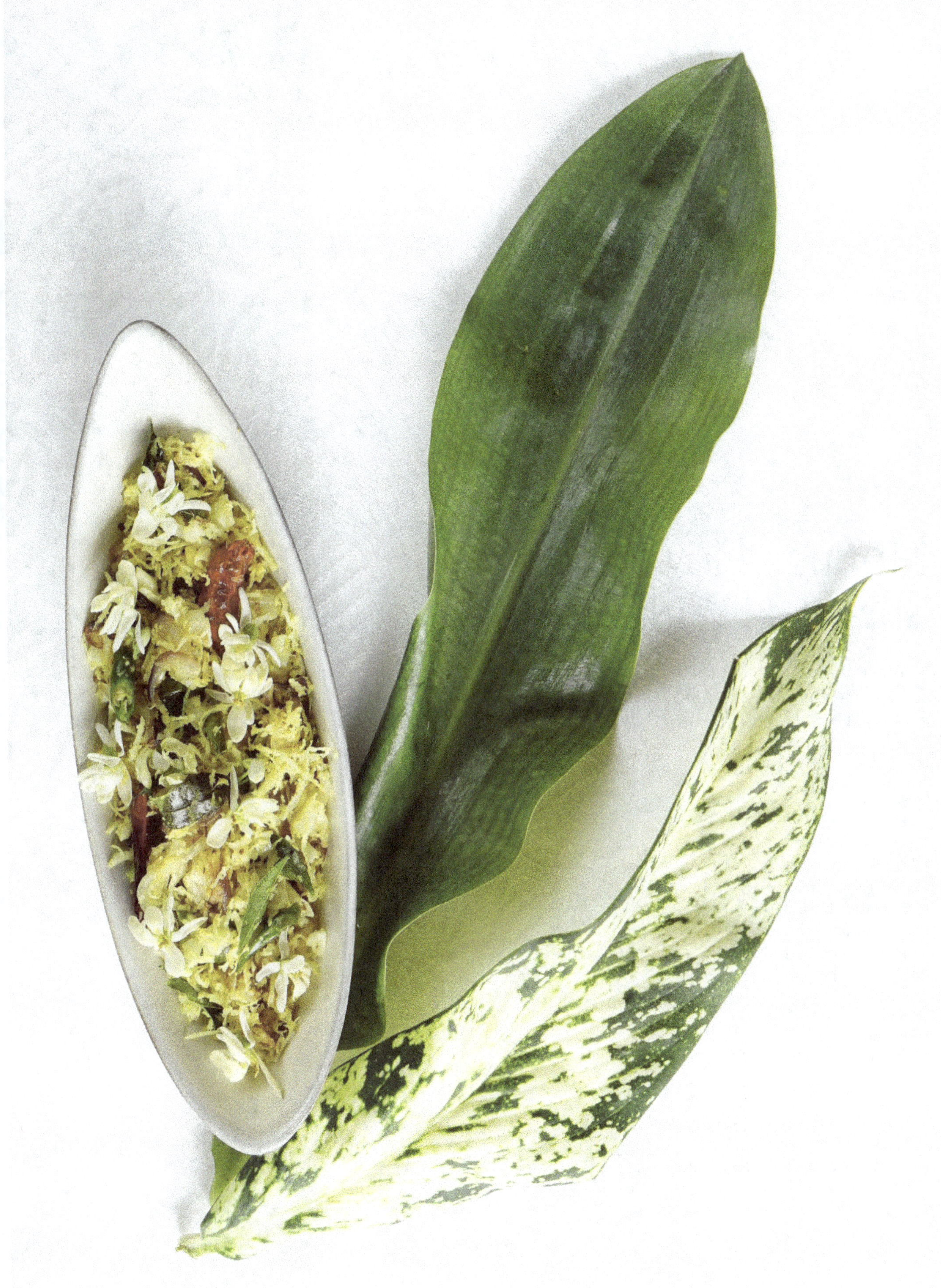

Moringa Flowers Stir-Fried With Eggs

A simple but substantial dish that's high in protein.
Serve this with hot steamed rice and some pickles
for a meal you'd want to eat every day.

Ingredients

1-2 cups moringa flowers
3 eggs
2 tbsp oil
1 tsp *bengal gram* (chickpeas)
1 tsp *urad dal* (black gram split)
1 big onion, finely chopped
2-3 green chillies, finely chopped
2-3 stalks curry leaves

Method

1. Heat oil in a pan.
2. Add mustard seeds, *bengal gram*, *urad dal*, green
   chillies, and chopped onion.
3. Sauté until golden brown.
4. Add moringa flowers and sauté for a few more
   minutes.
5. Add eggs and stir-fry for 2-3 minutes, or until
   the eggs are cooked through.
6. Add curry leaves and salt and pepper to taste.

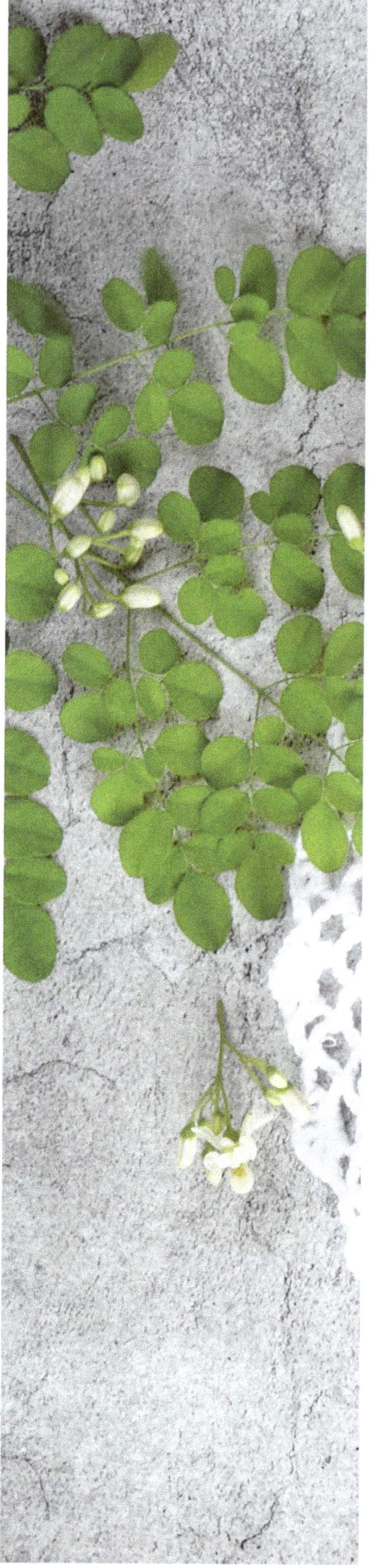

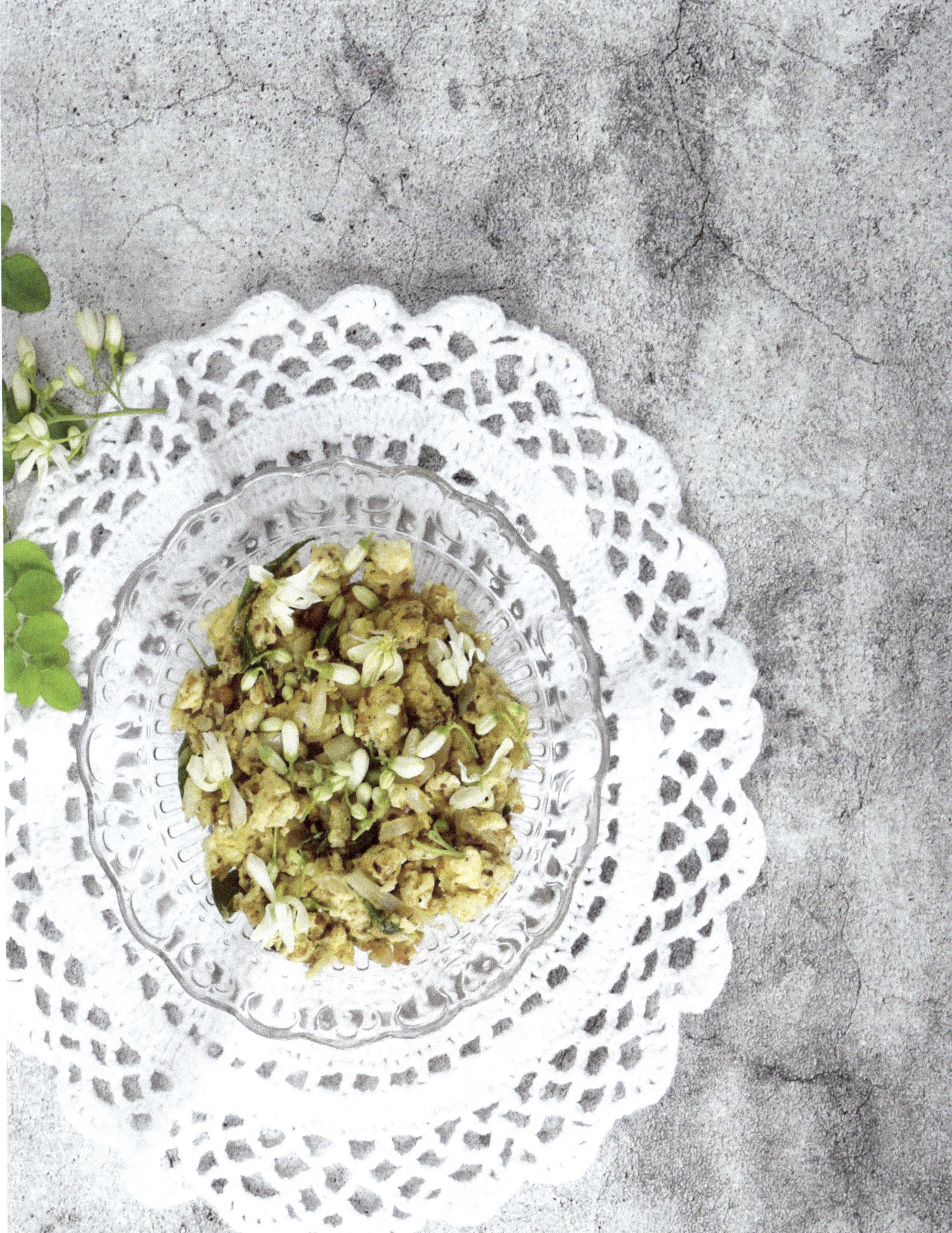

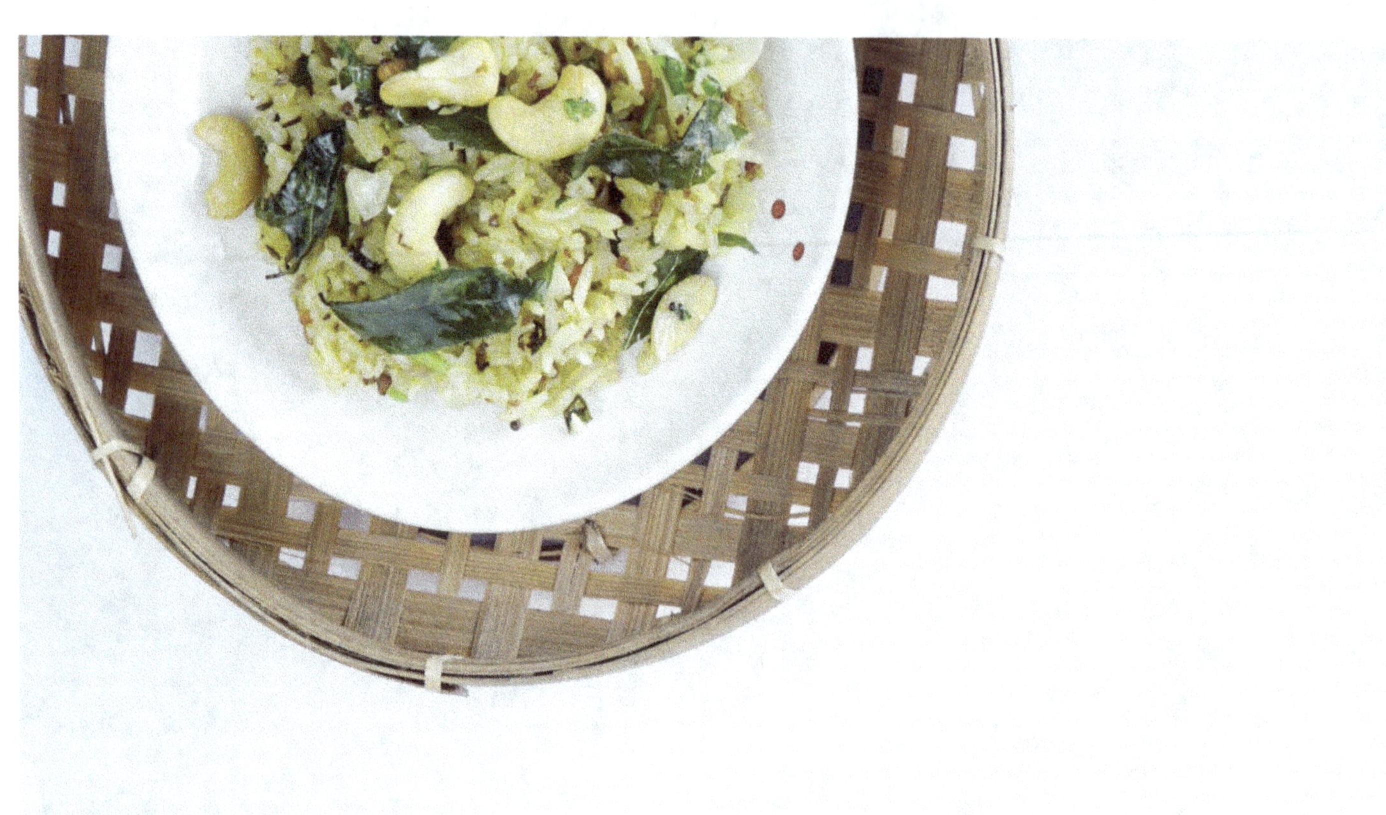
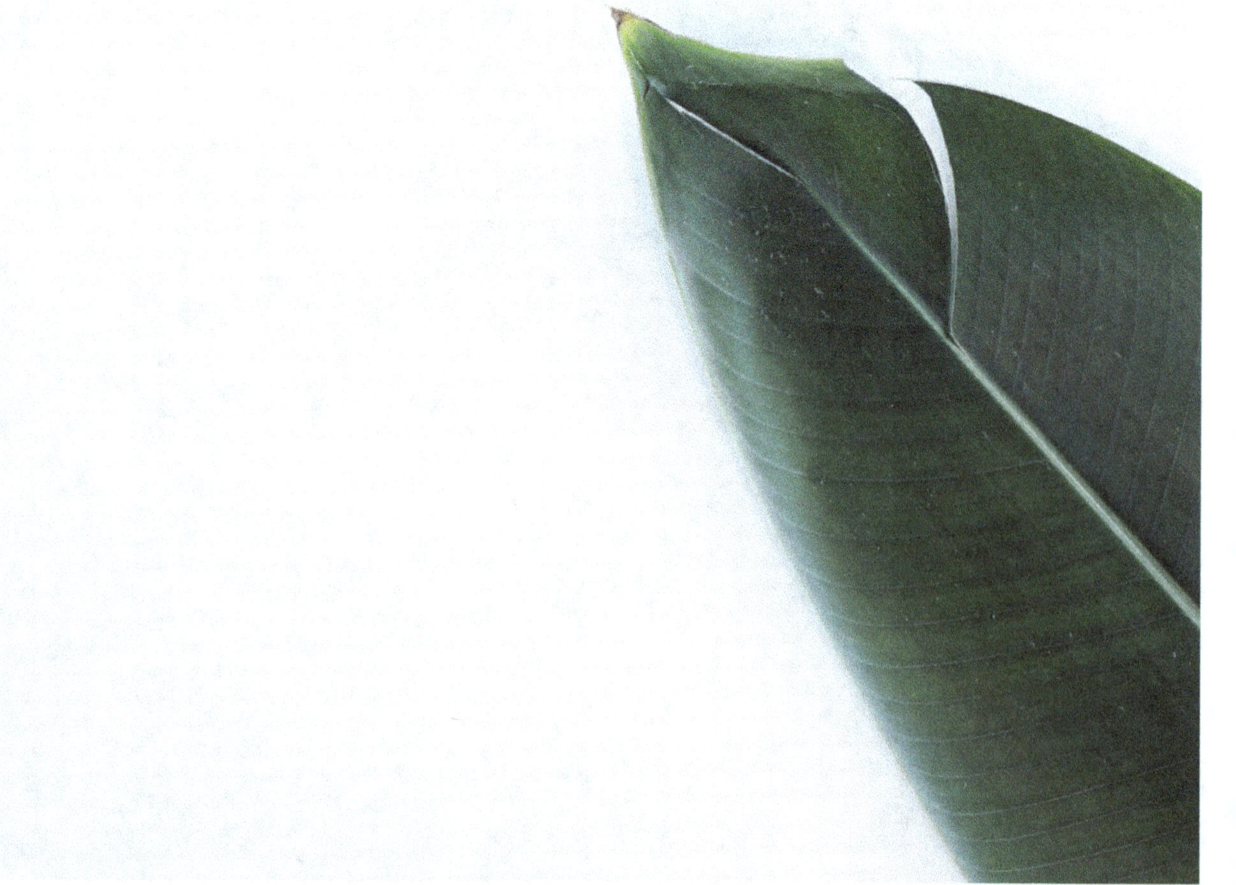

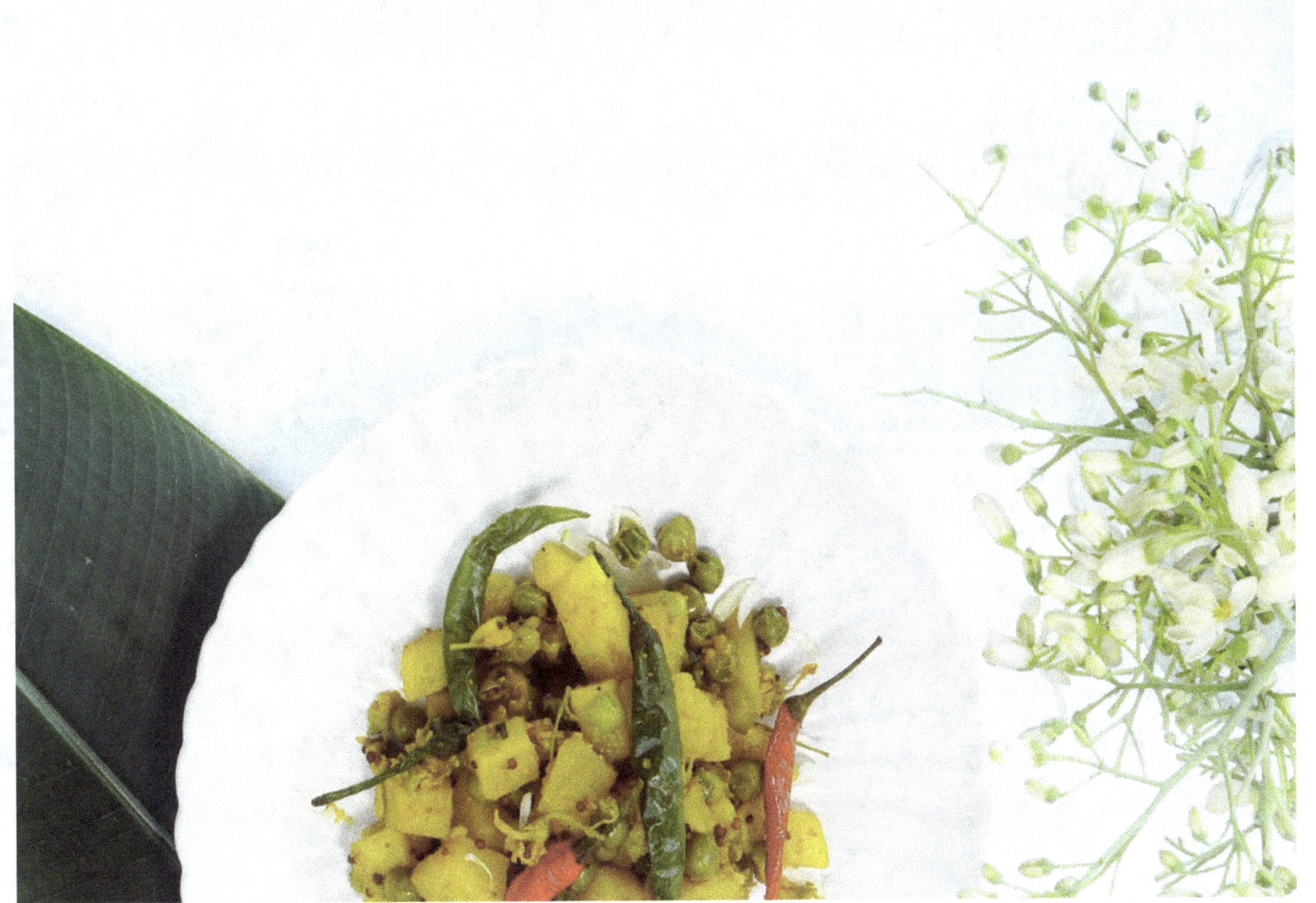

"In my food world, there is no fear
or guilt, only joy and balance.
So no ingredients is ever off-limits"
- Ellie Krieger

Bengali-Style Moringa Flower Curry With Potatoes

Those who love potatoes will adore this dish. It has a beautiful balance of spices and is packed with flavour.

Ingredients
2 cups moringa flowers
1 large potato, cut into small cubes
2 ½ tsp poppy seeds paste
2 ½ tsp mustard seeds paste
1 tsp cumin powder
1 tsp coriander powder
1 ½ tsp turmeric powder
1 tsp red chilli powder
Salt to taste
Water as required
2-3 tbsp mustard oil

Method
1. Heat oil in a frying pan. Add the cubed potatoes and sauté for 2 minutes.
2. Add salt and all the spices (cumin powder, coriander powder, red chilli powder, and turmeric powder) and stir for a few seconds.
3. Add the poppy seeds paste and mustard seeds paste.
4. Add a little water and cook for 2-3 minutes, stirring frequently.
5. Add the flowers.
6. Cover the pan and cook over low flame for 2-3 minutes.
7. Remove the lid, stir continuously for a few minutes until potato is soft.
8. Serve hot with plain rice.

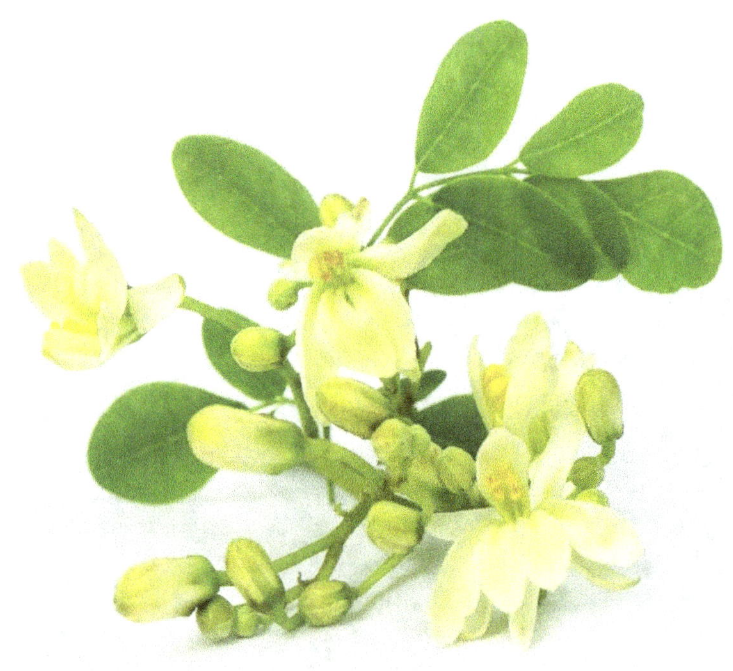

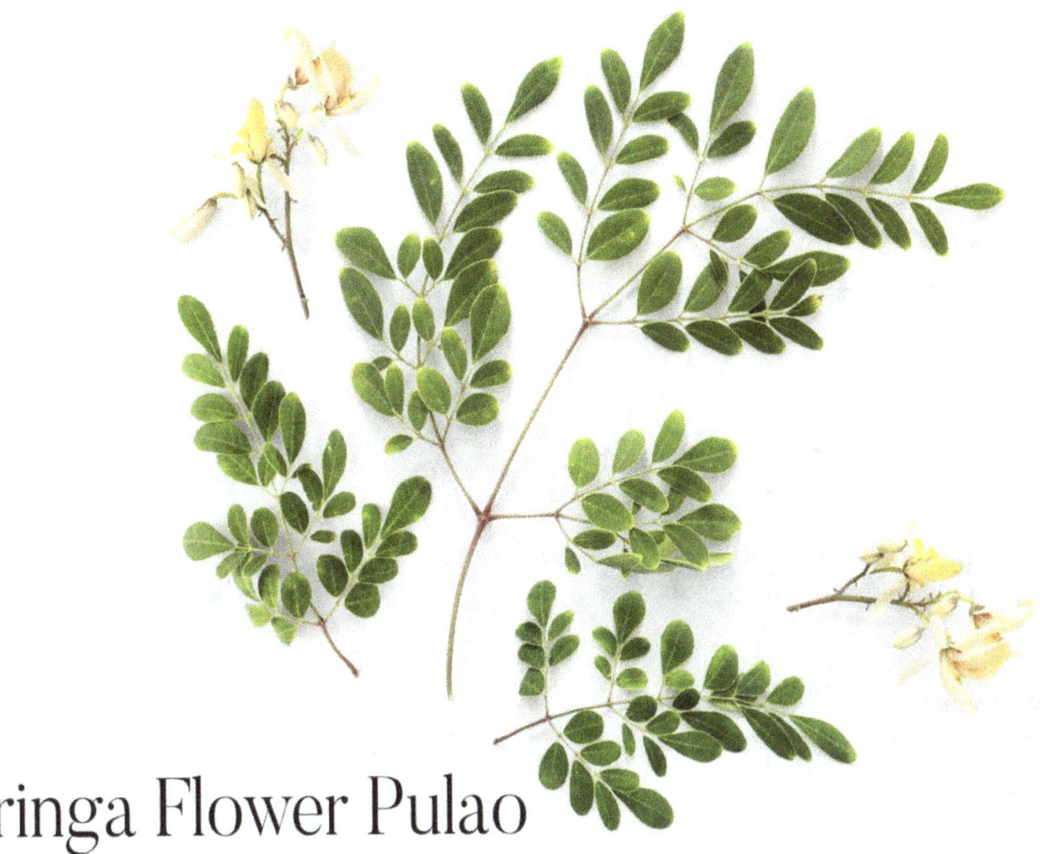

Moringa Flower Pulao

A wholesome dish that can be a meal on its own, or
serve with sides of papadums and pickles for extra kick.

Ingredients

2 tbsp oil
1 cup cooked rice*
1 tsp fennel seeds
1 tsp mustard seeds
1 tbsp *chana dal*
2 green chilies
6-8 cashew nuts
1 tsp chopped ginger
1 tsp chopped garlic
1 stalk curry leaves
1 onion, chopped
2 cups moringa flowers
¼ tsp turmeric flowers
½ tsp garam masala powder
½ tsp fennel seed powder
Salt to taste
½ cup fresh coriander leaves (for
garnishing)

** For best texture, make sure the rice
has cooled down first. You can also use
leftover rice that has been kept in the
refrigerator overnight.*

Method

1. Heat oil in a pan.
2. When hot, add fennel seeds,
   mustard seeds and *chana dal*, and
   let it splutter.
3. Add green chillies, chopped
   ginger, and garlic.
4. Sauté for a few seconds.
5. Add cashew nuts and curry
   leaves.
6. Cook till the cashews turn golden
   brown.
7. Add the onions and sauté till
   glossy.
8. Add the moringa flowers and
   sauté on low flame for about 5
   minutes.
9. Add salt, turmeric powder, fennel
   powder, and garam masala. Fry
   for another 2 minutes.
10. Add the cooked rice.
11. Mix well, and garnish with
    coriander leaves to serve.

Moringa Flower Fritters

These crispy, crunchy delights are delicious and packed
with nutrients. Serve as a starter, side dish, or snack.

Ingredients
1 cup moringa flowers
1 cup gram flour
8-10 garlic cloves
2-3 green chillies
1 small onion, chopped
2 tbsp fresh coriander leaves, chopped
Salt to taste
Water as required
Oil for shallow frying

How to prepare the flowers for cooking
1. Separate the flowers from the soft branches.
2. Remove the stems.
3. Soak in water and salt for at least 10 minutes.
4. Rinse, then refill the water and salt and soak
   for another 10 minutes.
5. Rinse again and pat dry.

Method
1. Wash the flowers thoroughly and chop them up
   coarsely.
2. Make a paste with the garlic and green chillies.
3. Add gram flour and the garlic-green chillies paste
   in a bowl.
4. Add just enough water to make a thick batter.
5. Add the chopped flowers, onions, and coriander.
6. Add salt to taste.
7. Heat oil in a pan.
8. Drop the batter into the oil, one spoonful at a time.
9. Fry at medium heat for about a minute.
10. Flip them over and continue frying until they turn
    a golden shade.
11. Serve hot with a dipping sauce of your choice.

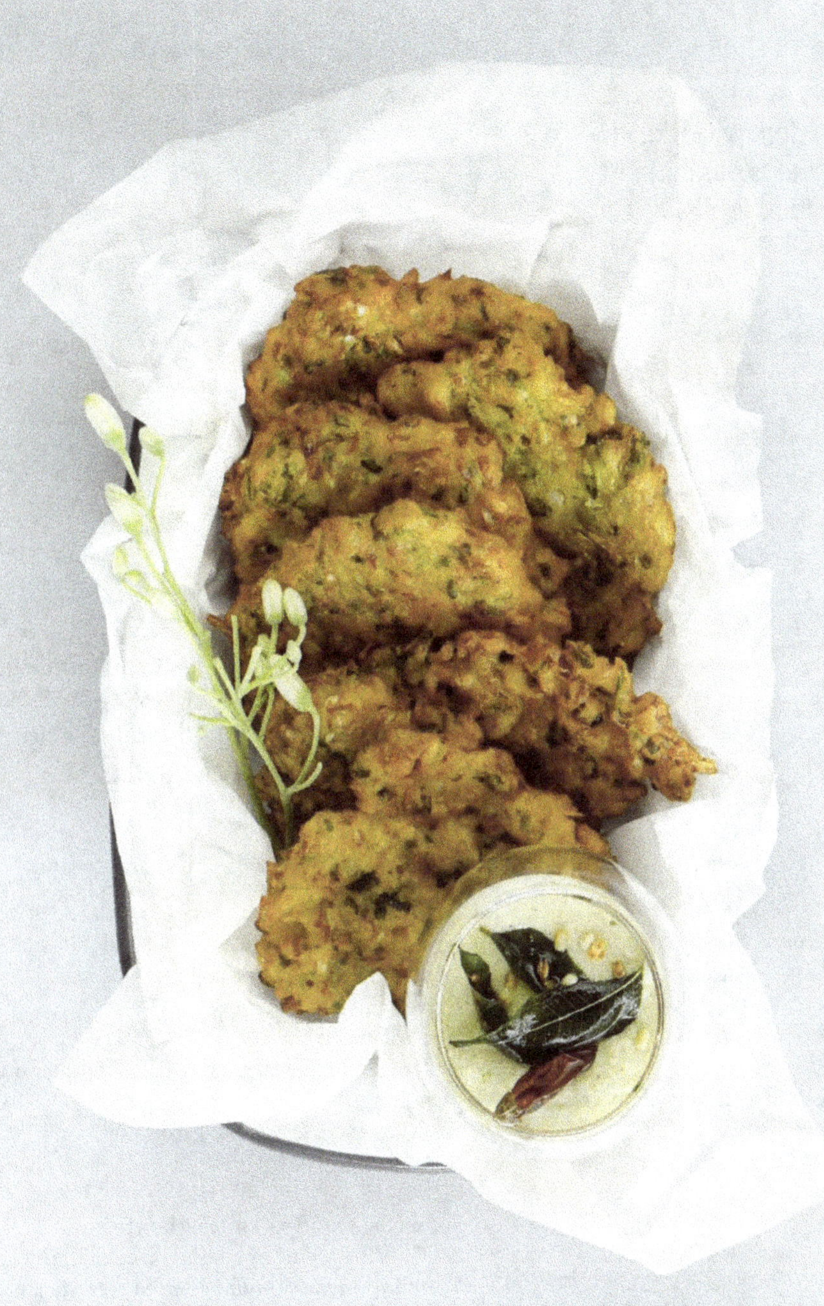

Moringa Flower Chutney

This flavourful chutney that will take any dish to the next level and is particularly enjoyable as a dip for fried foods.

Ingredients
1/4 cup fresh moringa flowers
3-4 green chillies
½ cup mint leaves
2 stalks curry leaves
¼ cup freshly grated coconut
2 cloves garlic
½ tsp grated ginger
Salt to taste
2 tsp lemon juice

For tempering
2 tsp oil
½ tsp *urad dal*
½ tsp cumin seeds
½ tsp mustard seeds
¼ tsp *asafoetida**
1 stalk of curry leaves
5-6 moringa flowers
1 tbsp water

**This is a gum that's derived from a type of fennel. It has a strong garlic-like aroma and when added to dishes, lends a robust savoury flavour.*

Method (to grind)
1. Place all chutney ingredients in a blender and blitz into a fine paste.
2. Add salt and lemon juice to taste.
3. Pour into a dish and set aside.

Method (to temper)
1. Heat oil in a small pan.
2. Add *urad dal*, seeds, and *asafoetida*, and allow to splutter.
3. Add curry leaves, moringa flowers, and water.
4. While still sizzling, pour the mixture onto the chutney and stir gently.
5. Serve as a dip or an accompaniment to meals.

Moringa Flower Raita

Add a zesty lift to any meal by pairing it with a side of this raita. It will taste even better if you chill it in the refrigerator for 20-30 minutes before serving.

Ingredients
1 cup curds (yogurt)
½ cup boiled moringa flowers
Salt to taste
Water as needed
1 green chilli, finely chopped
Pinch of grated ginger
Sautéed cumin powder and red chilli powder (for garnishing)
Fresh coriander leaves (for garnishing)

Method
1. Add the yogurt to a mixing bowl.
2. Dilute the yogurt by adding water a little bit at a time until you achieve your preferred consistency.
3. Squeeze the moringa flowers and let the flowers cool down before adding to the yogurt.
4. Add salt, chopped green chili, and grated ginger, and mix well.
5. Sprinkle with sautéed cumin powder, chilli powder, and coriander leaves.

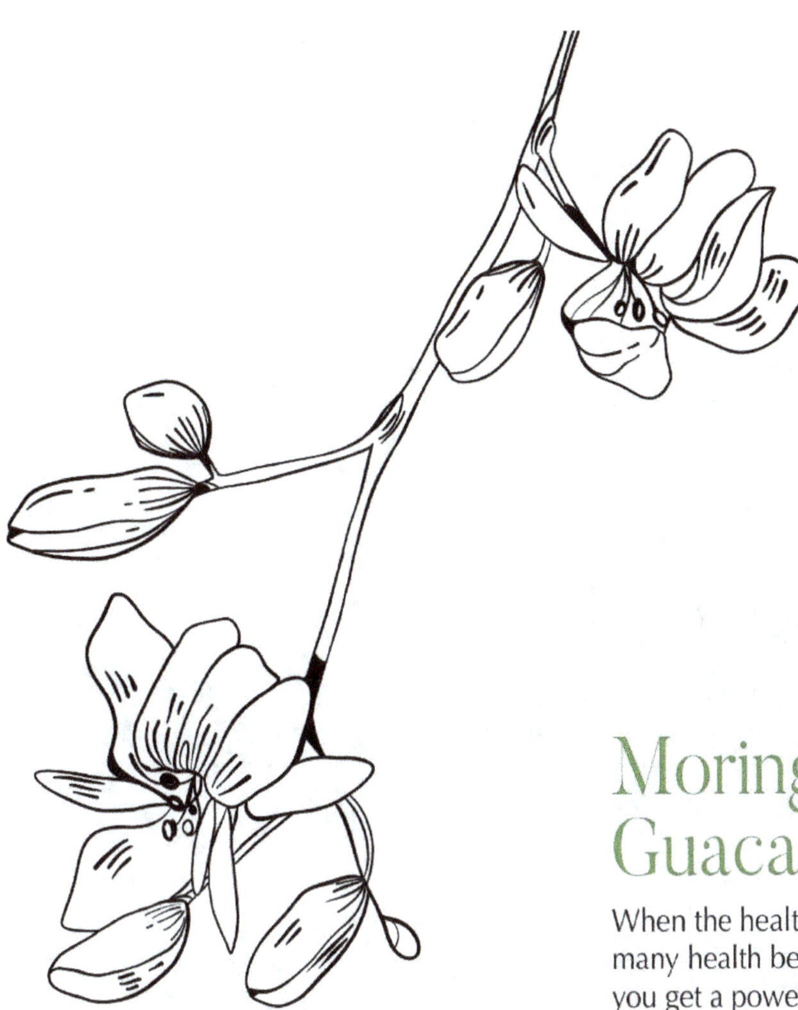

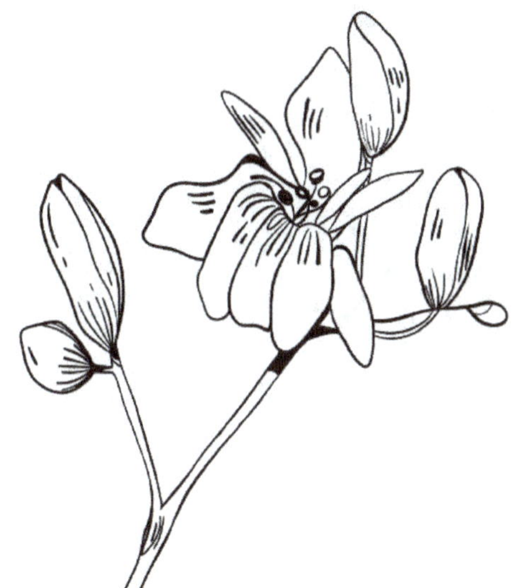

Moringa Flower Guacamole

When the healthy fats of the avocado meet the many health benefits of the moringa flowers, you get a powerhouse of nutrients.

Ingredients

1 clove garlic
½ jalapeño or red chilli, seeded
2 avocados
½ cup moringa flowers, boiled
¼ small onion, peeled and chopped
1 small tomato
Juice of one lime
Salt to taste

Method

1. Place the garlic, onion, and jalapeño or red chilli in a food processor. Blend until the ingredients are finely chopped.
2. Cut tomato into quarters.
3. Add tomato wedges to the mix. Pulse until the tomato is coarsely chopped
4. Pour the mixture into a bowl.
5. Add avocado flesh to the mixture.
6. Add lime juice and boiled moringa flowers.
7. Season with salt.
8. Mash the ingredients with a fork until everything is combined but still chunky.
9. Serve immediately with chips, crackers, or vegetable sticks.

Moringa Flower Cutlets

These moreish morsels make for delightful tea time treats.
You can also sandwich them between soft buns to make
vegetarian sliders.

Ingredients
1 cup fresh moringa flowers
3 potatoes
1 onion, chopped
2 tbsp chopped fresh coriander leaves
1 green chilli, chopped
1 tsp cumin powder
1 tsp chilli flakes
2 tsp black pepper powder
Salt to taste
2 tsp vinegar
Water for boiling
Oil for shallow frying

Method
1. Boil a small pot of water and add vinegar to it.
2. Add the flowers and boil for 5 minutes.
3. Drain the water. Set the flowers aside.
4. Boil the potato. Once they are cooked through, drain
   the water and let cool for a while.
5. Peel the skin and mash the potatoes.
6. Transfer the flowers and mashed potatoes into a
   mixing bowl. Add all the remaining ingredients and
   mix well.
7. Grease your palm with a bit of cooking oil. Scoop
   about a tablespoon of the mixture onto your palm
   and shape into balls. Flatten lightly.
8. Add a little oil to the griddle.
9. Pan fry the cutlets on both sides until brown.
10. Serve hot with Moringa Flower Chutney or Moringa
    Flower Raita (pg 54).

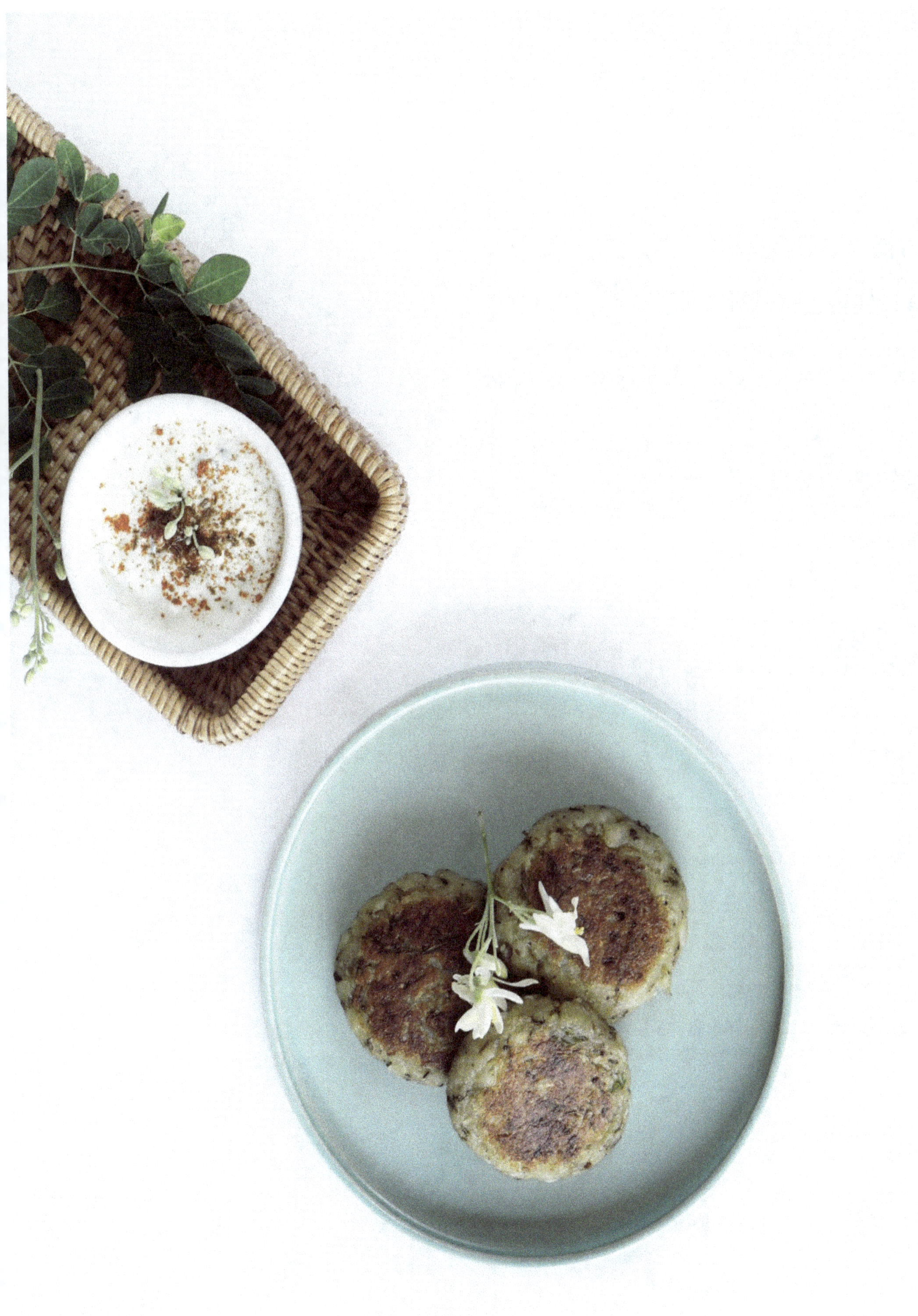

Moringa Flower Buds With Minced Chicken

The buds add a tender texture that pair well with the chicken. If you can't get enough buds, you can replace them with young moringa flowers.

Ingredients
2-3 cups moringa flower buds
½ cup oil
½ cup garlic
½ cup spring onions
500gm minced chicken
2 tomatoes
1 tsp cumin powder
½ tsp turmeric powder
2 tsp coriander seeds, crushed
1 ½ tsp red chilli powder
½ cup yogurt
Salt to taste
3-4 green chillies, chopped
Garam masala
Coriander leaves for garnishing

Method
1. Boil moringa buds for five minutes.
2. Turn off flame.
3. Leave for an hour.
4. Strain the buds and rinse.
5. Squeeze out excess water and set the buds aside.
6. In a frying pan, heat up ¼ cup oil.
7. Add green garlic and spring onions, and sauté for a few minutes.
8. Add minced chicken and cook for a few minutes.
9. Add chopped tomato, cumin powder, turmeric powder, coriander seeds, and chilli powder.
10. Cook for a few minutes.
11. Add moringa buds and yogurt.
12. Add salt to taste.
13. Add chopped green chillies.
14. Cook until the chicken is done.
15. Add garam masala.
16. Garnish with coriander leaves and serve hot with rice or roti.

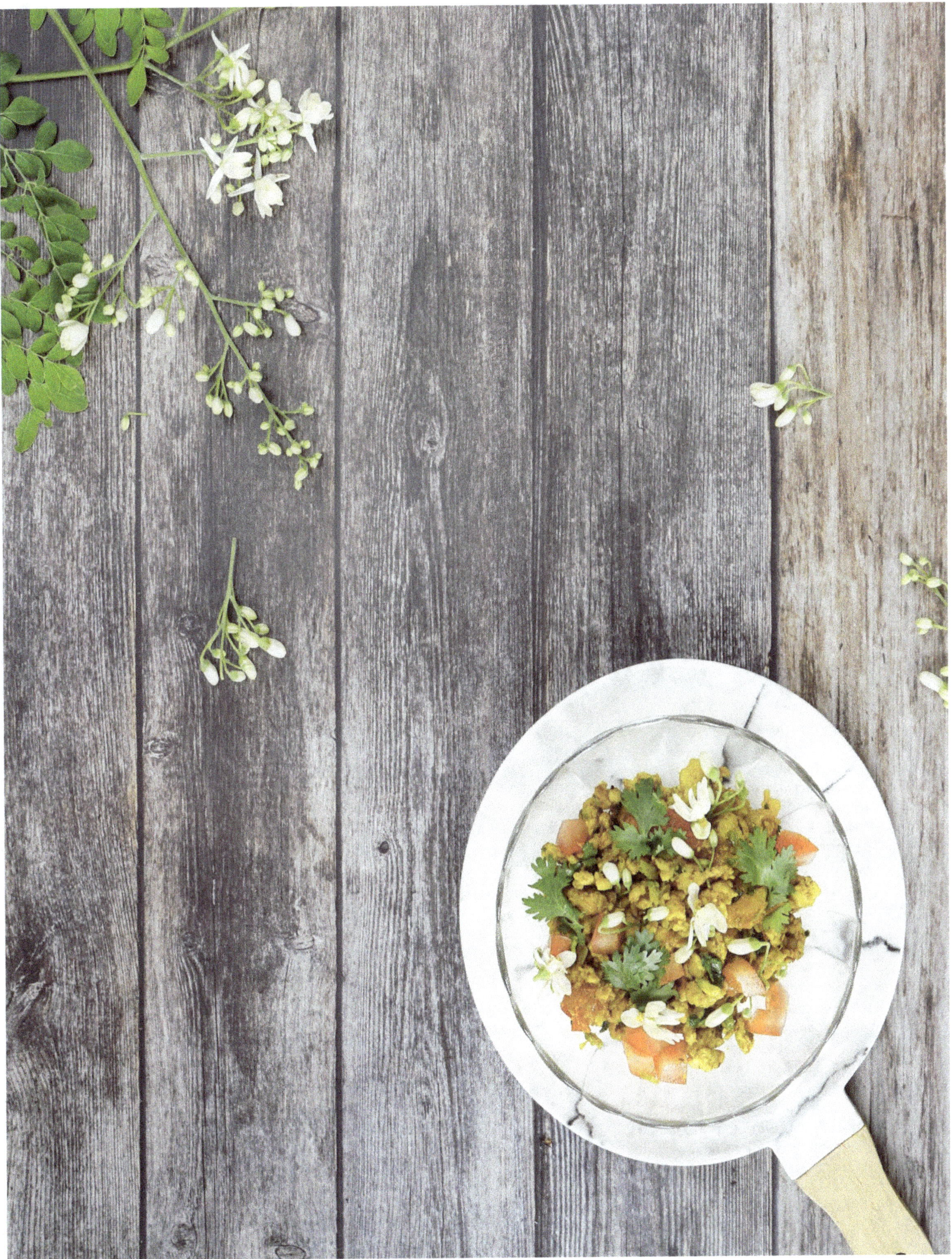

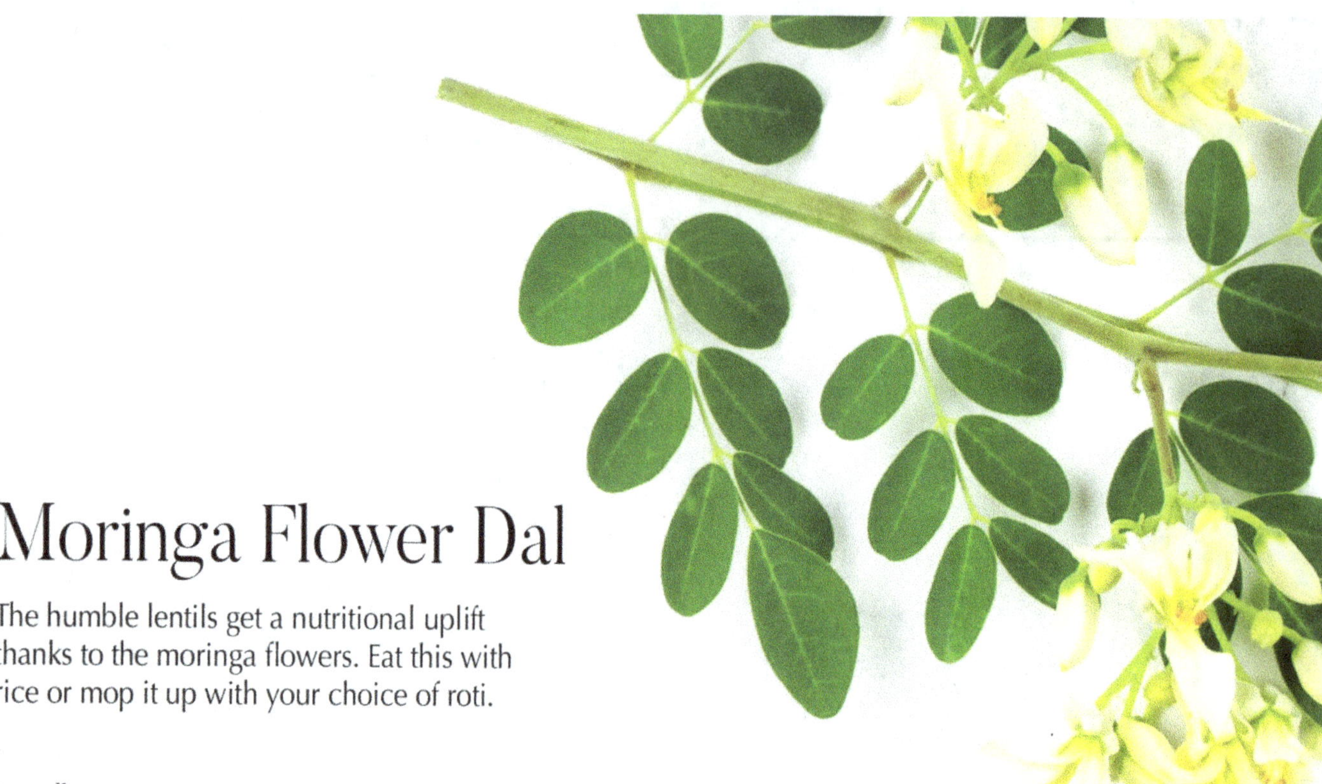

Moringa Flower Dal

The humble lentils get a nutritional uplift
thanks to the moringa flowers. Eat this with
rice or mop it up with your choice of roti.

Ingredients

3 cups moringa flowers
1 cup *chana dal/gram dal* (soak overnight)
I medium onion
1 medium tomato
2 tbsp freshly grated or desiccated coconut
Salt to taste

Tempering

2 tsp oil/butter
½ tsp mustard seeds
¼ tsp *asafoetida*
¼ tsp turmeric powder
6-7 green chillies
1 stalk curry leaves

Method

1. Cook the *chana dal* until they soften.
2. Heat up a pan and add oil.
3. Add mustard seeds, *asafoetida*, and curry leaves,
   and allow to splutter.
4. Add green chillies and sauté for a minute.
5. Add onions and sauté until translucent.
6. Add tomatoes and cook until soft and the oil
   separates.
7. Add coconut and sauté for a few minutes.
8. Add moringa flowers and sauté well.
9. Cover and cook for 8-10 minutes.
10. Add cooked dal and salt to taste.
11. Add water as required (depending on how thin or
    thick you want the dal to be).
12. Let simmer for another 10 minutes.
13. Remove from heat and serve with hot rice.

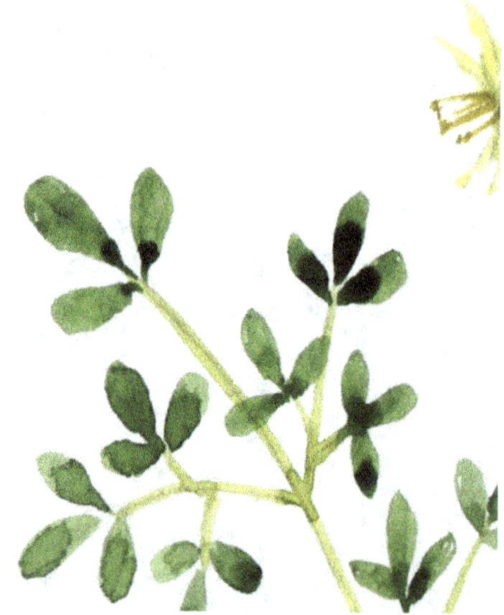

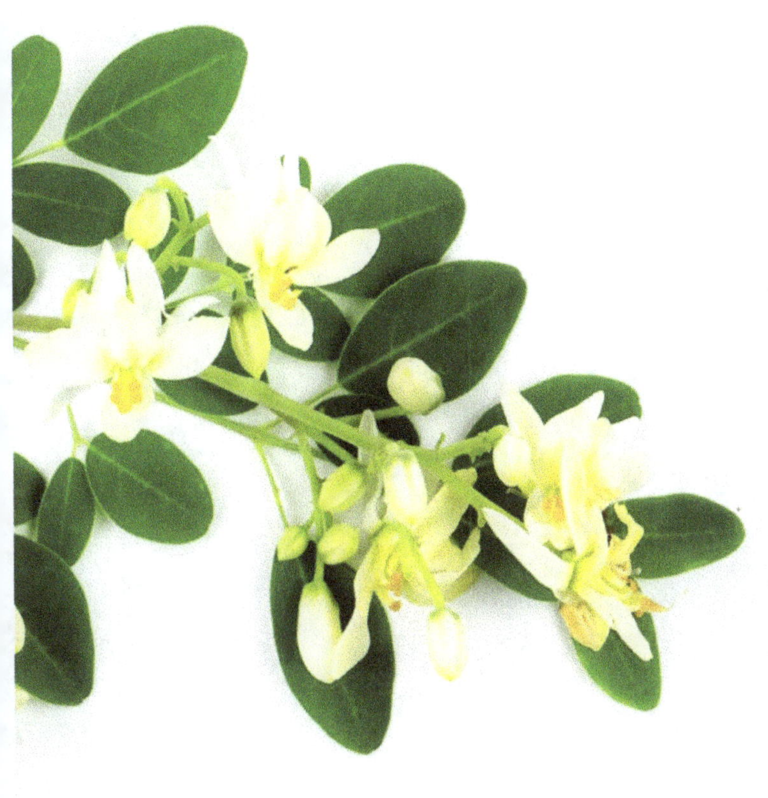

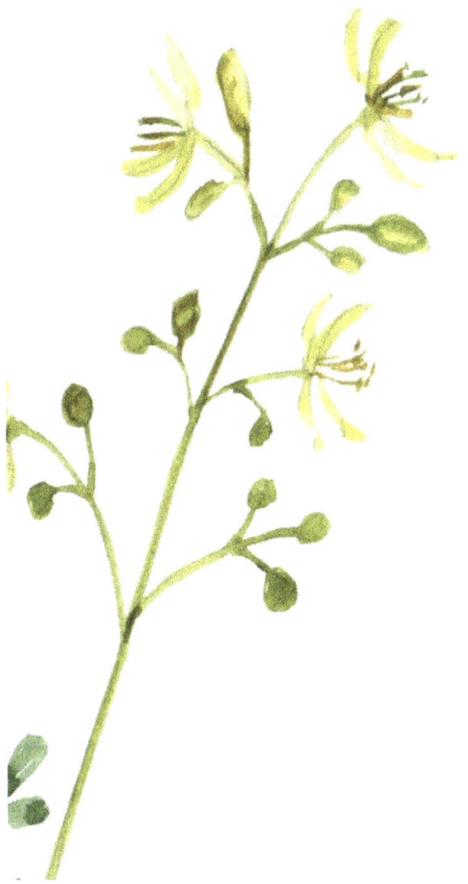

Moringa Flower Soup

A simple and healthy soup that's great for the whole family.

Ingredients
1 cup moringa flowers
1-inch stick of cinnamon
5-6 shallots, chopped
2 pods with cloves
1 tomato, chopped
Black pepper and salt to taste
2-3 tsp oil or clarified butter (ghee)
Water as required
1 tsp corn flour
Fresh coriander leaves (for garnishing)

Method
1. In a pan, add oil or ghee. Once it gets hot, add cloves and cinnamon.
2. Add shallots and garlic, and sauté for a few minutes.
3. Add the flowers and sauté for a minute.
4. Add the chopped tomato and 2 glasses of water. Boil for a few minutes.
5. Add salt to taste. Boil for 5-6 minutes.
6. Remove the cloves and cinnamon.
7. In a bowl, add corn flour with a little bit of water to make a slurry.
8. Add to the soup and mix well to let it thicken.
9. Add black pepper to taste, and garnish with fresh coriander. Serve hot.

Moringa Flower Dosa

This thin South Indian pancake is light yet fulfilling, and goes well with any chutneys and curries.

Ingredients
½ cup uncooked rice
1 cup moringa flowers
1 tbsp freshly grated coconut
5-7 red chillies
1 big onion, chopped
1 tsp tamarind, soaked in a little water
Salt to taste
Oil for frying

Method
1. Soak the rice in water for half an hour. Drain and place in a blender.
2. Add the freshly grated coconut, red chillies, and tamarind water, and blend into a coarse consistency.
3. Add the chopped onion and flowers. Season with salt.
4. Heat up a griddle.
5. With a ladle, pour the batter onto the griddle and spread it out in a circular shape.
6. Add a teaspoon of oil around the dosa and fry on both sides over medium flame.
7. Serve hot with chutney, dal, or curry.

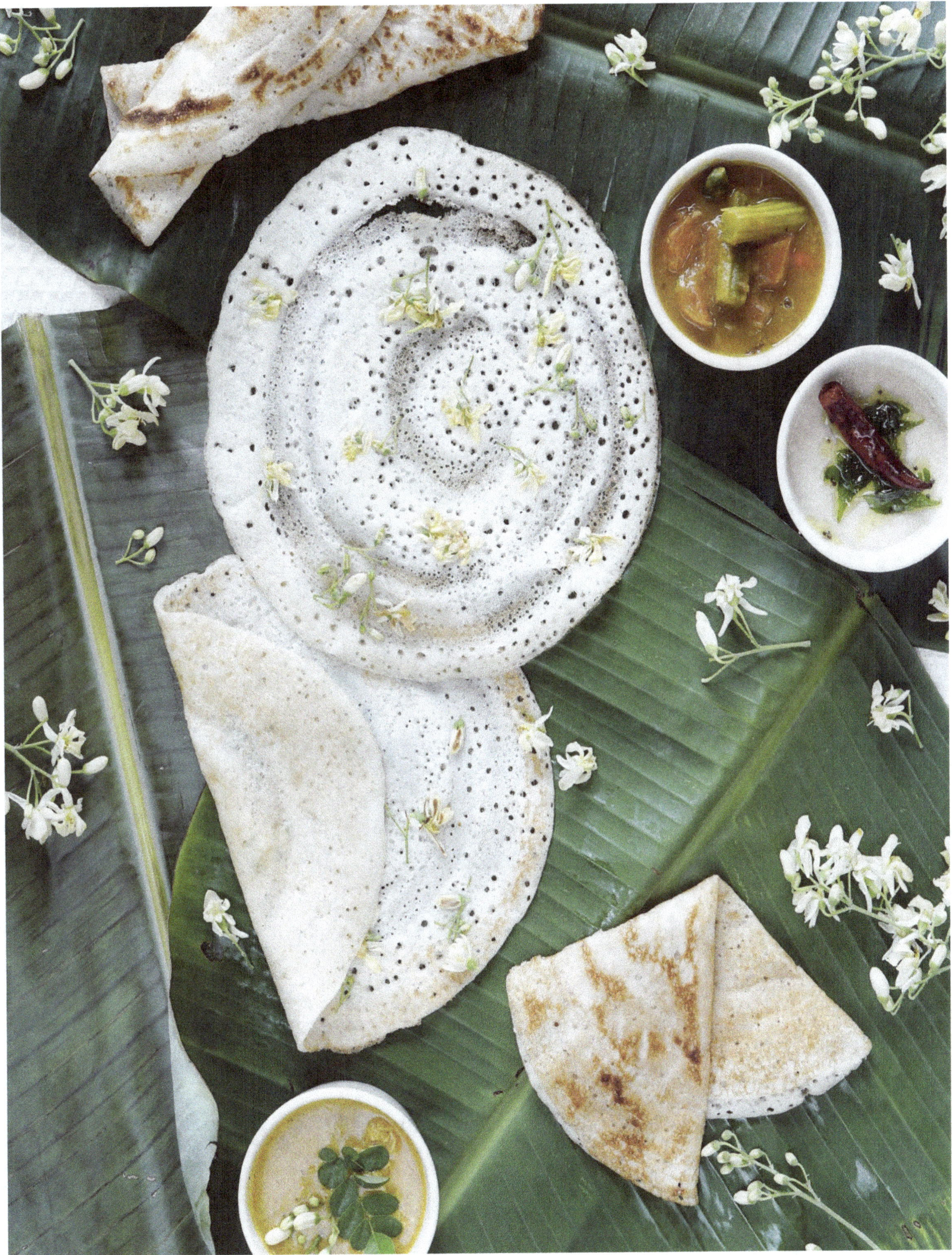

Moringa Flower Kheer

A creamy dessert that's easy to enjoy. Children will love this!

Ingredients
1 cup moringa flowers
1 tbsp powdered sugar
1 cardamom pod, crushed
1 cup boiled milk
½ cup water
¼ tsp ghee

Method
1. Add milk, water, cardamom pod, and the flowers into a small pot.
2. Boil the mixture over medium flame until it is half reduced. Stir in between.
3. Add sugar and let it boil for the another 5 minutes on low flame.
4. Transfer to a bowl.
5. Add few drops of ghee and serve.

Tip For a bit of crunch, top with nuts that have been roasted in ghee.

Moringa Flower Masala Milk

A tad spicy, a little bit sweet, and a whole lot of comfort in a hot mug. This is a great way to enjoy the benefits of the moringa flowers and quench your thirst at the same time.

Ingredients
1 cup moringa flowers
½ cup water
1 cup milk
Crushed pepper
Pinch of turmeric powder
¼ tsp crushed cardamom
⅛ tsp crushed pepper
1 tbsp palm candy

Method
1. Add the flowers and water to a pot and boil until cooked or most of the water has evaporated.
2. Add milk, turmeric powder, crushed pepper, crushed cardamom, and palm candy.
3. Keep the flame low and boil for 2-3 minutes.
4. Strain and pour into cups to serve. You can also let it cool down and chill before serving as a cold beverage.

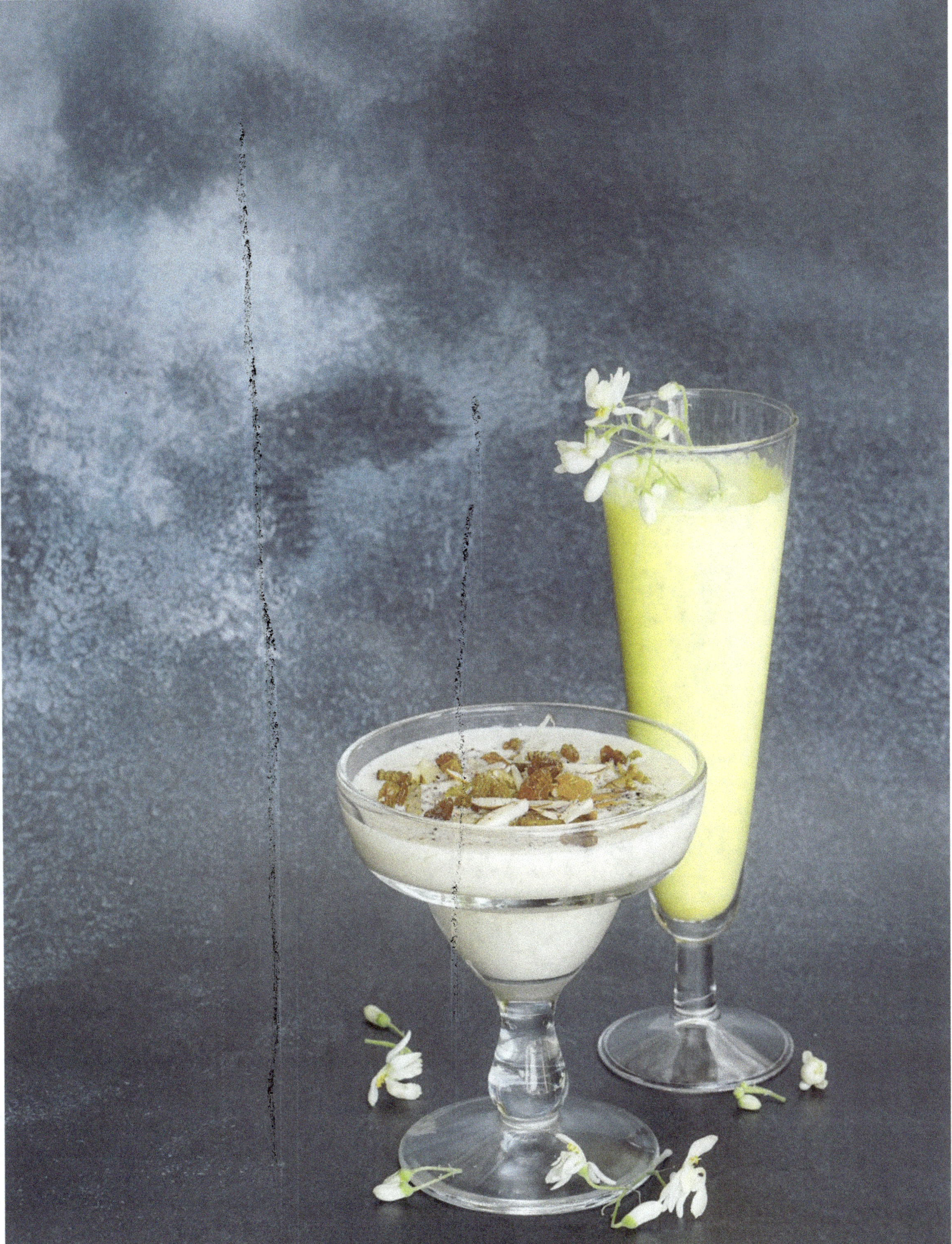

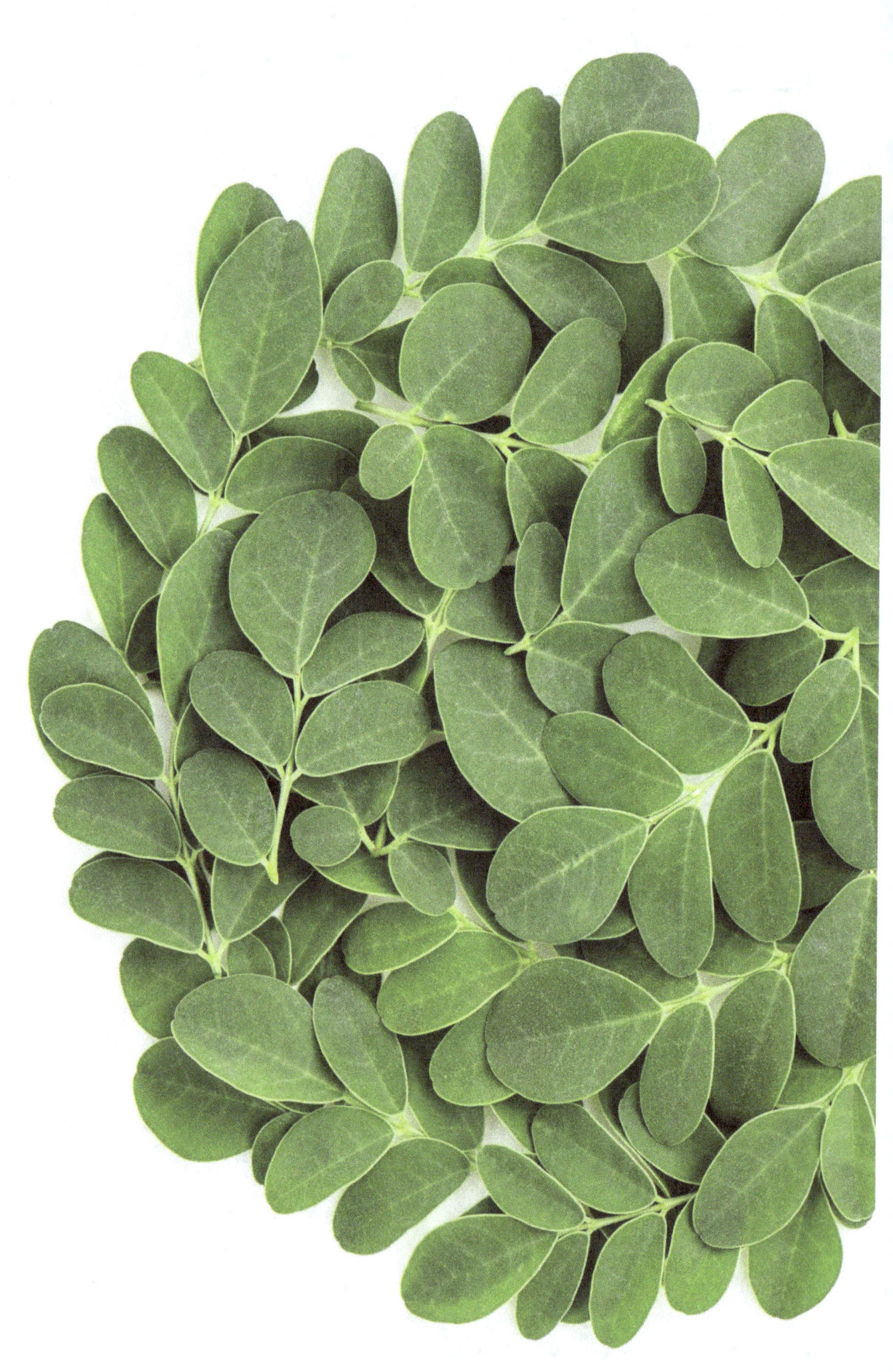

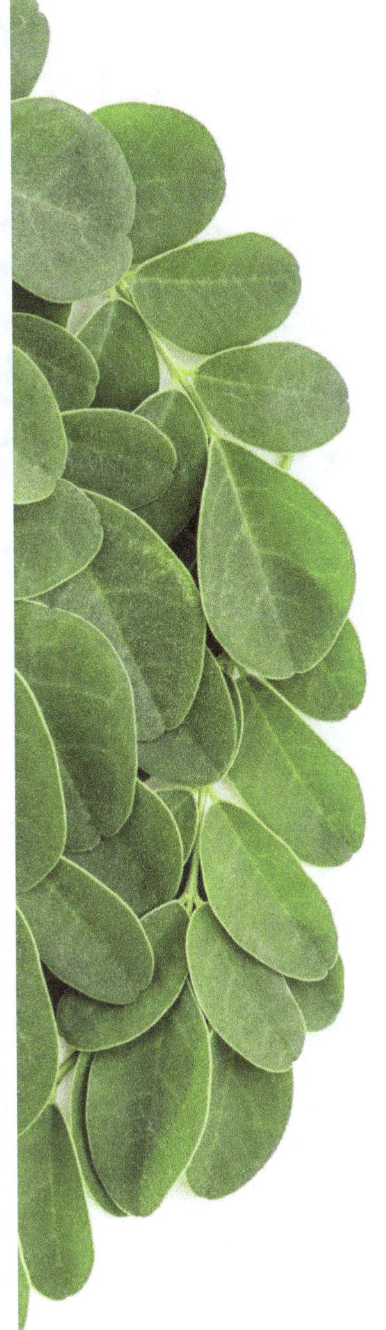

MORINGA LEAVES

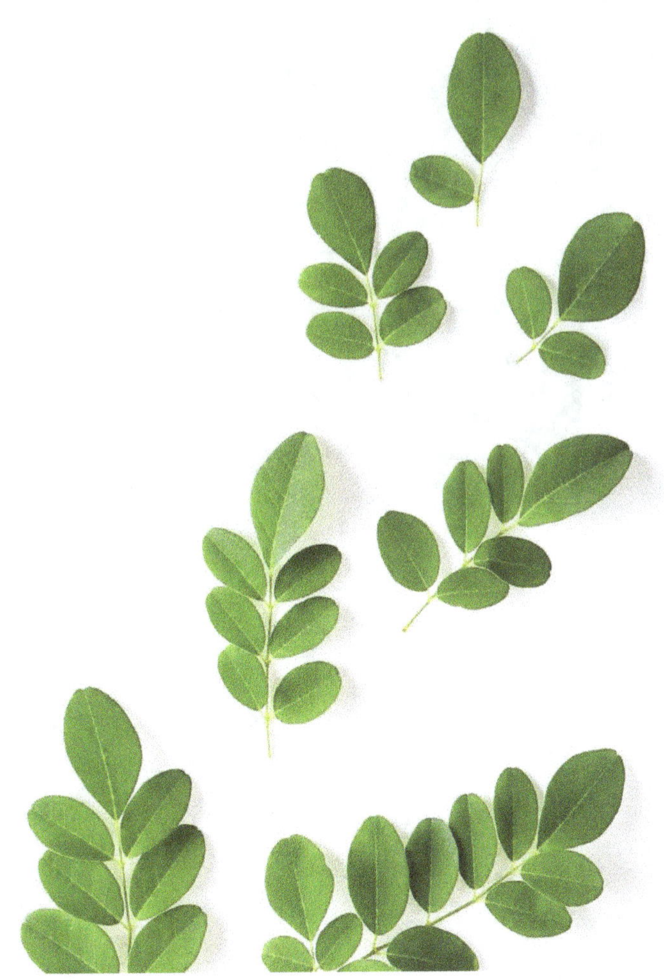

5 THINGS TO KNOW ABOUT MORINGA LEAVES

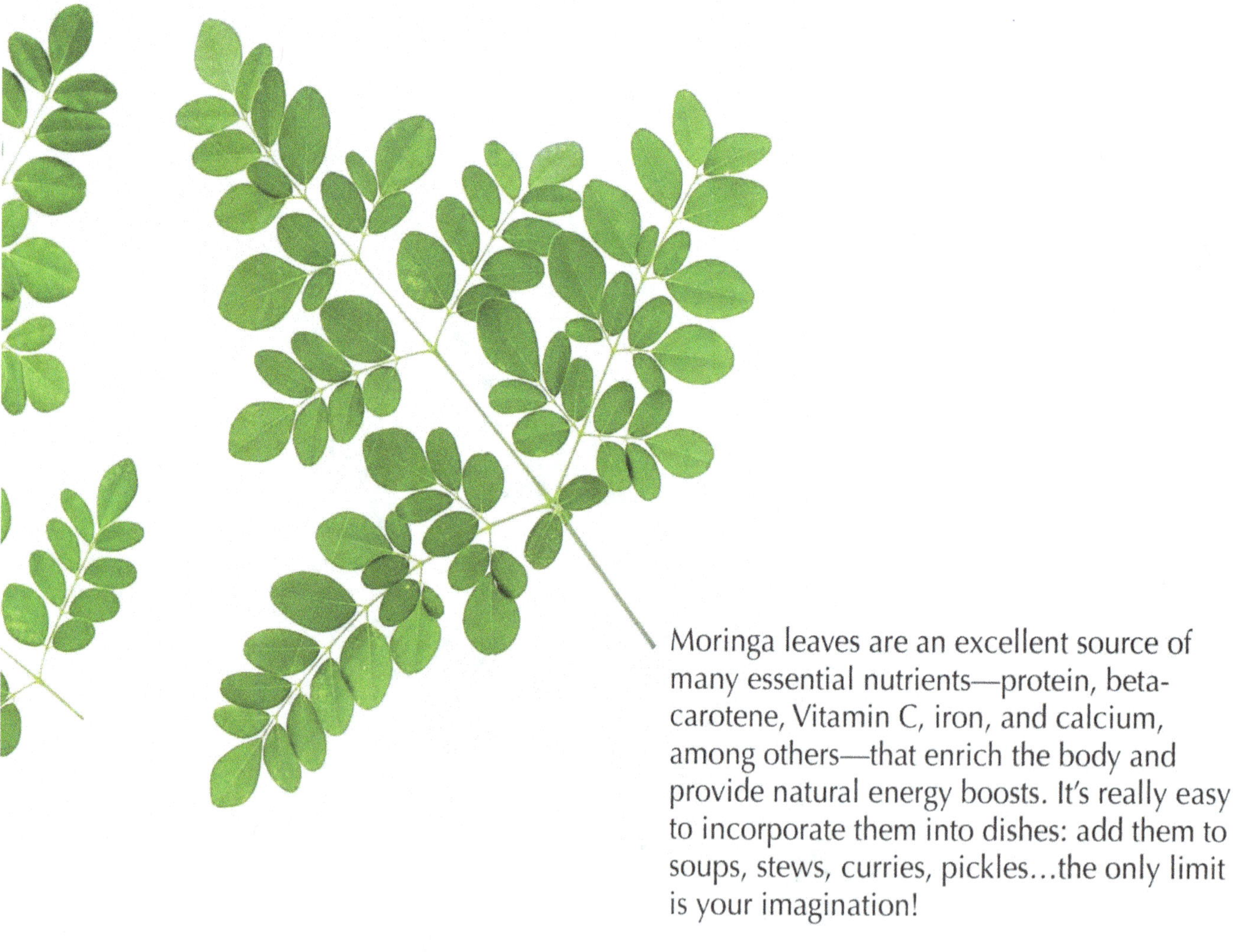

Moringa leaves are an excellent source of many essential nutrients—protein, beta-carotene, Vitamin C, iron, and calcium, among others—that enrich the body and provide natural energy boosts. It's really easy to incorporate them into dishes: add them to soups, stews, curries, pickles…the only limit is your imagination!

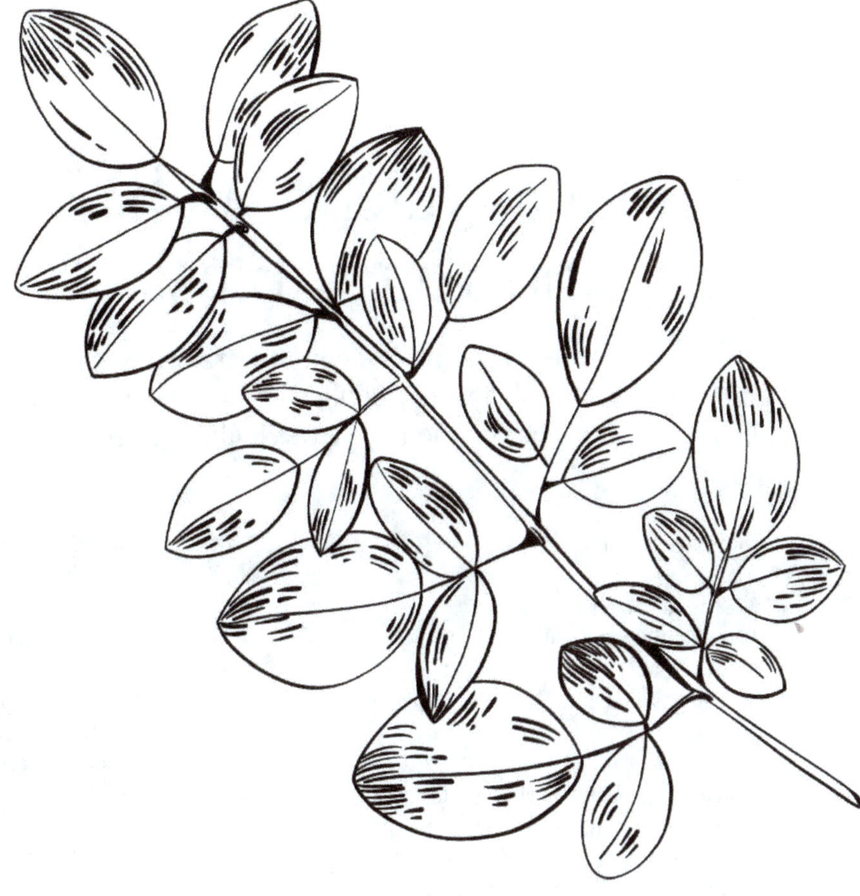

#1

Unlike some other parts of the tree, you don't have to wait for the leaves to ripen. In fact, they are best eaten as young shoots or growing tips as the older they get, the tougher they become.

#2

To prepare the leaves, remove them from the branches or stems (these do not soften even with cooking and therefore, are not suitable to be eaten) first and wash before adding to dishes.

#3

The leaves can be slightly chewy when first cooked and may even have traces of bitterness, but once cooked through, they give off a wonderful hearty flavour.

#4

An easy way to approach cooking moringa leaves is to use them as you would spinach. You can simply steam them for a few minutes until they soften, then season with salt or sauté with shallots or garlic. Avoid overcooking or you risk losing its nutrients.

#5

The leaves can also be baked into breads and pastries to add colour and a healthy twist to your breakfast and teatime staples.

POWDER VS LEAVES: A CONVERSION GUIDE

For all the recipes in this book, you can substitute fresh moringa leaves for moringa powder and vice-versa. Just follow this simple equation:

2 cups of fresh moringa leaves =
2-3 tbsp/about 40gm moringa powder

Moringa Quiche With Feta And Vegetables

This classic French tart—one of the most versatile dishes around as you can make it with a variety of fillings—is more wholesome and nutritious when you add moringa leaves to the recipe.

Ingredients (pie crust)

1 large egg
2 ½ tbsp ice water
1 ½ cups all-purpose flour
½ tsp sea salt
10 tbsp unsalted butter, cut into small cubes

Method

1. In a small mixing bowl, whisk together the egg and ice water. Set the bowl aside.
2. Add flour and salt to a food processor and pulse for a few minutes until mixed through.
3. Add the butter and blitz until the mixture takes on the texture of coarse meal.
4. Add the egg and ice water. Pulse again until dough forms.
5. Transfer the dough onto a lightly-floured board and roll it out into a circle, following the dimensions of your quiche pan or dish.
6. Lay the dough onto the quiche pan and press the dough into place. Use a firm but gentle pressure.
7. Trim off any dough that's hanging over the rim of the pan or dish.
8. Chill the pan or dish with the dough in the freezer for 20-30 minutes.
9. When ready to bake, remove from the freezer and pour in the filling. (Tip: a cold crust will give a flaky texture after baking!)

Ingredients (filling)

1 tbsp butter
1 medium onion, diced
1 tbsp garlic, minced
½ cup mushroom, diced
½ cup bell pepper of your choice, diced
2 cups moringa leaves
1 medium carrots, shredded
4 eggs
1 cup milk
½ cup feta cheese
Salt and pepper to taste
¼ cup shredded cheese of your choice

Method

1. Pre-heat oven to 350°F/180°C
2. In a small pot or pan, melt butter over medium heat.
3. Sauté onions and garlic until fragrant.
4. Add mushrooms and bell peppers, and sauté for a few minutes.
5. Reduce heat.
6. Add the moringa leaves and shredded carrots. Sauté until leaves soften.
7. Remove vegetables from heat and mix in the feta cheese.
8. Pour the mixture into the pie crust.
9. Sprinkle salt and pepper to taste and mix through.
10. Whisk 4 eggs with 1 cup of milk. Add salt and pepper to taste.
11. Pour slowly over the vegetables in the crust.
12. Bake for about 20 minutes.
13. Remove from oven and add shredded cheese of your choice. Continue to bake for about 20-25 minutes or until the filling sets.
14. Allow to sit for 10-15 minutes before cutting and serving.

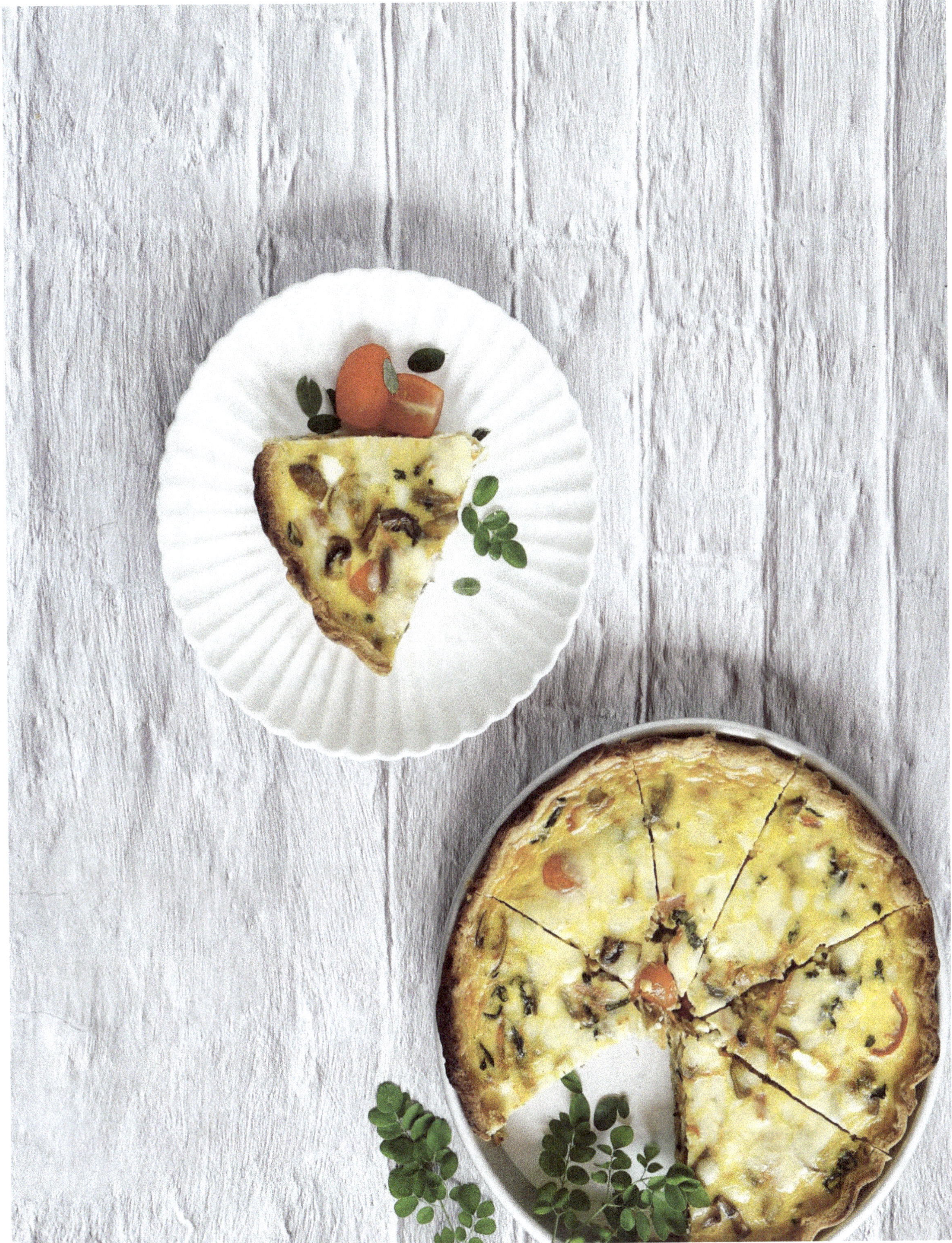

Pandesal Buns

This classic Filipino bread roll is popularly eaten for breakfast.
The name comes from the Spanish word meaning "salt bread"
and originated in the 16th century when the Spanish colonised
the Philippines. The addition of moringa leaves lends a slightly
nutty taste to the pillowy soft rolls.

Ingredients
1 cup moringa leaves
3 cups all-purpose flour
¼ cup sugar
1 tsp salt
1 medium egg
2 tbsp oil
1 cup lukewarm water
1 ½ tsp instant dry yeast
¼ cup fine bread crumbs

Method
1. Wash the moringa leaves, then pat them dry and chop coarsely.
2. In a large bowl, mix together flour, sugar, and salt.
3. Add the chopped moringa leaves and mix until well incorporated.
4. Make a well in the centre and add egg, oil, water, and instant dry yeast.
5. Mix until all the ingredients are well blended.
6. Lightly sprinkle a flat surface with flour.
7. Knead the dough until it becomes smooth and elastic.
8. Form dough into a ball. Lightly oil it and transfer to a clean, dry bowl.
9. Cover with a plastic wrap and let the dough rise until it doubles in size, or about 10-15 minutes.
10. Lightly punch the dough to release gas bubbles.
11. Place dough on a flat surface and divide into two.
12. Roll each dough into logs, then divide each log into 8 equal portions.
13. Roll each portion into small balls. Set aside.
14. Sprinkle the bread crumbs onto a flat surface.
15. Roll the balls in the bread crumbs until fully covered.
16. Arrange them on a baking sheet.
17. Cover, and let rise until they double up (about 20-30 minutes).
18. Preheat the oven to 350°F/185°C. Bake the buns for about 15 minutes or until they are evenly browned.
19. Enjoy the rolls with your favourite fruit jam or for a savoury twist, slap on some Moringa Pesto (pg 82).

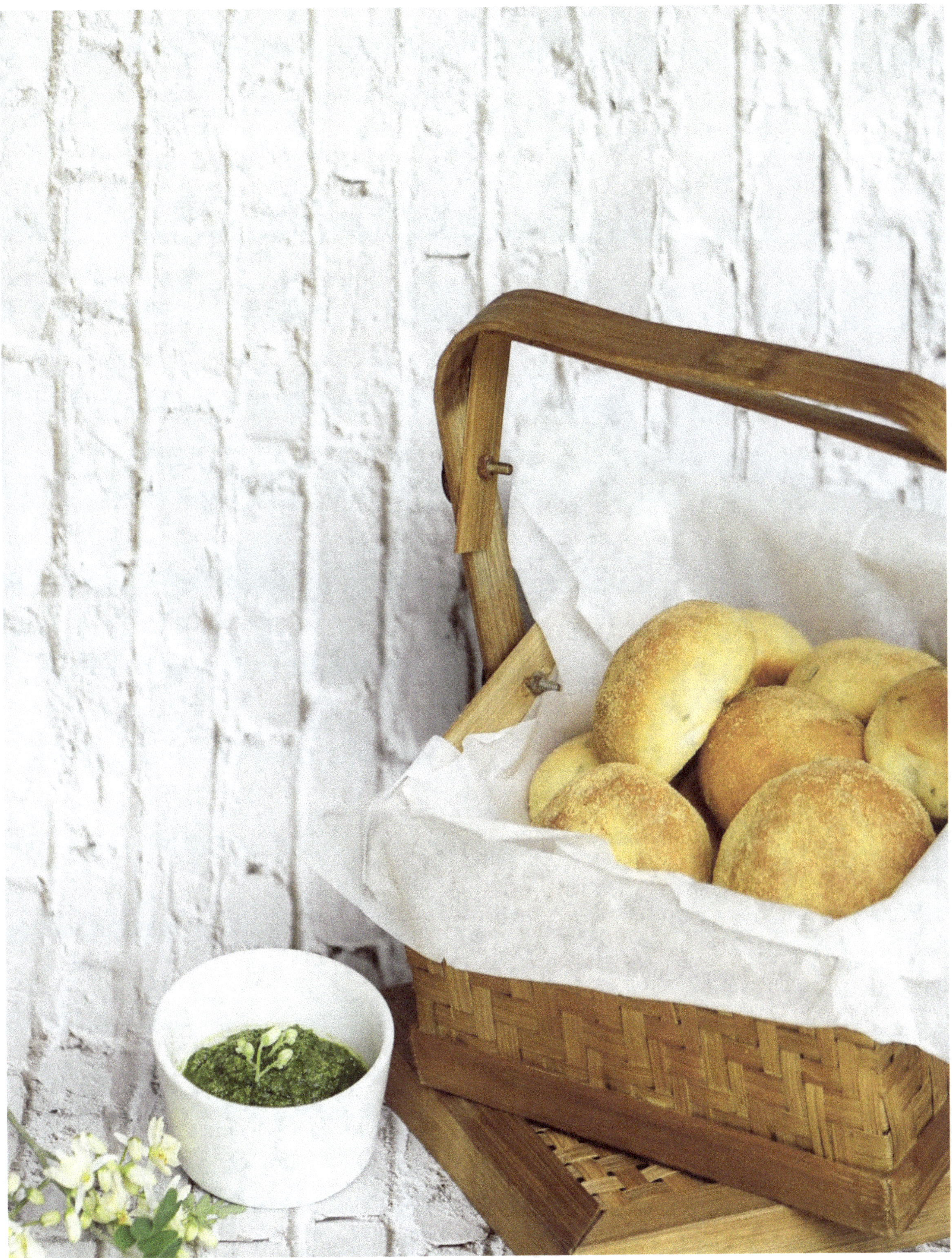

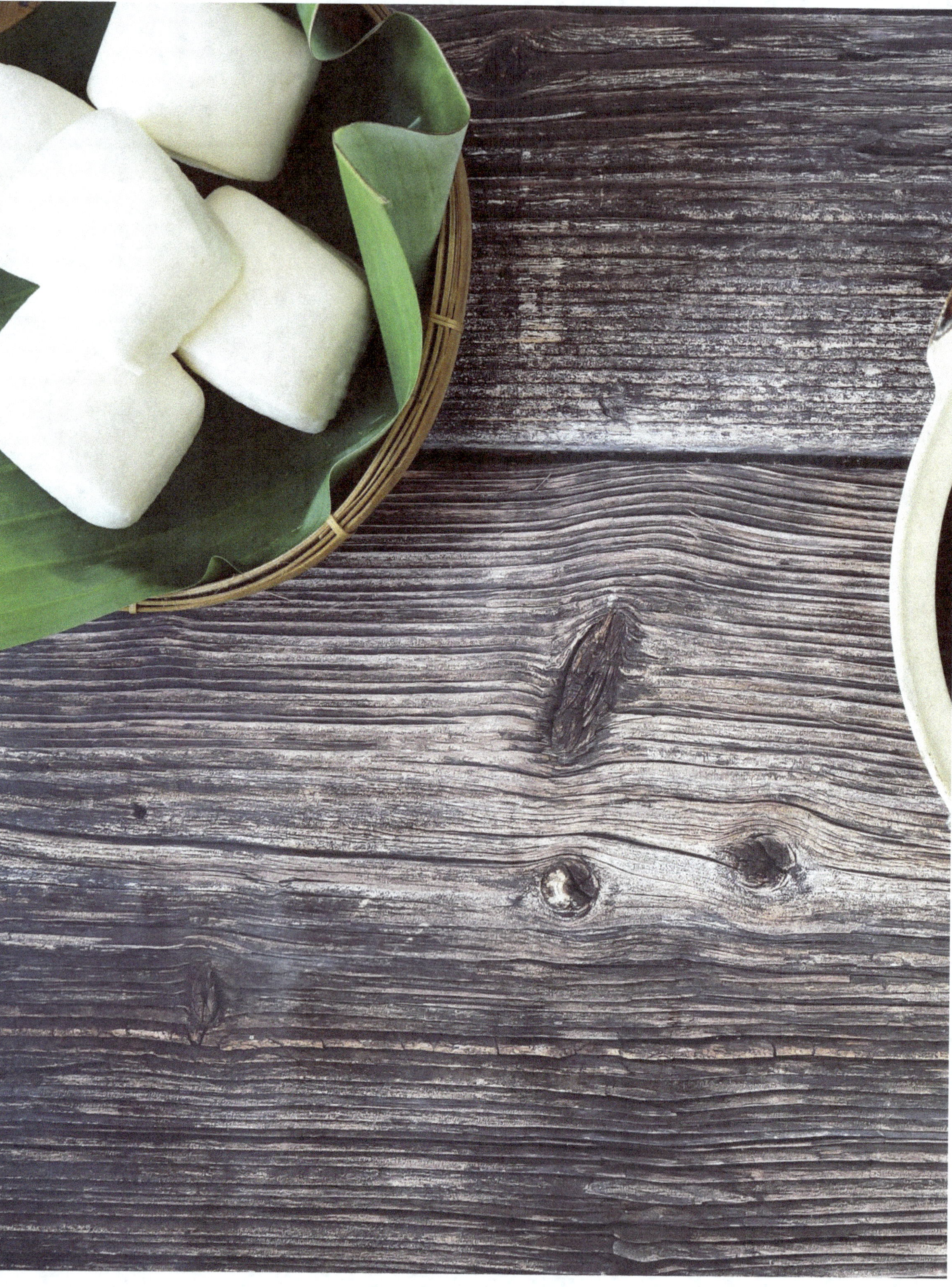

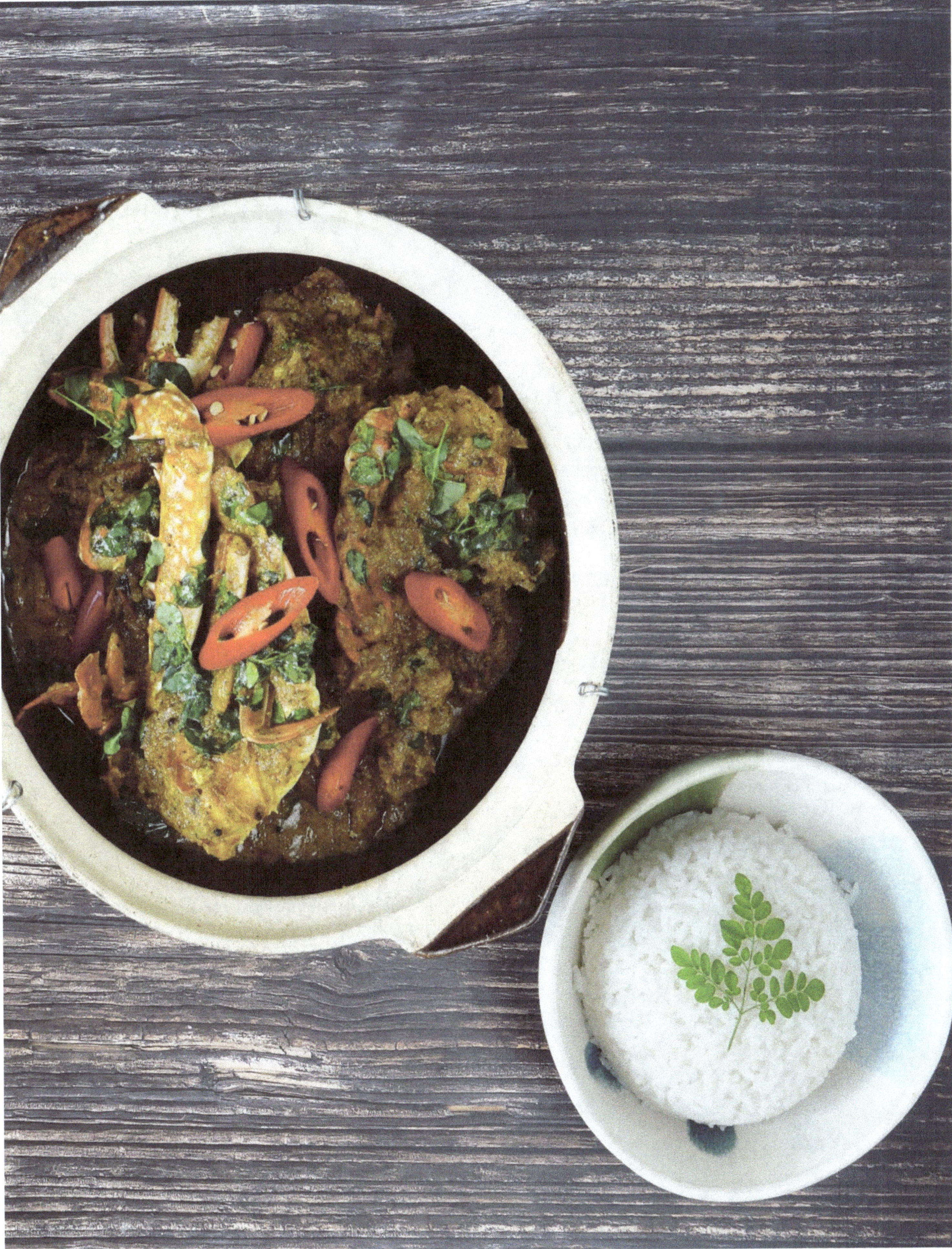

Crab Curry With Moringa

This finger-licking-good curry will have you reaching for a second helping of rice! It's just as ideal served with freshly steamed *mantou* or roti.

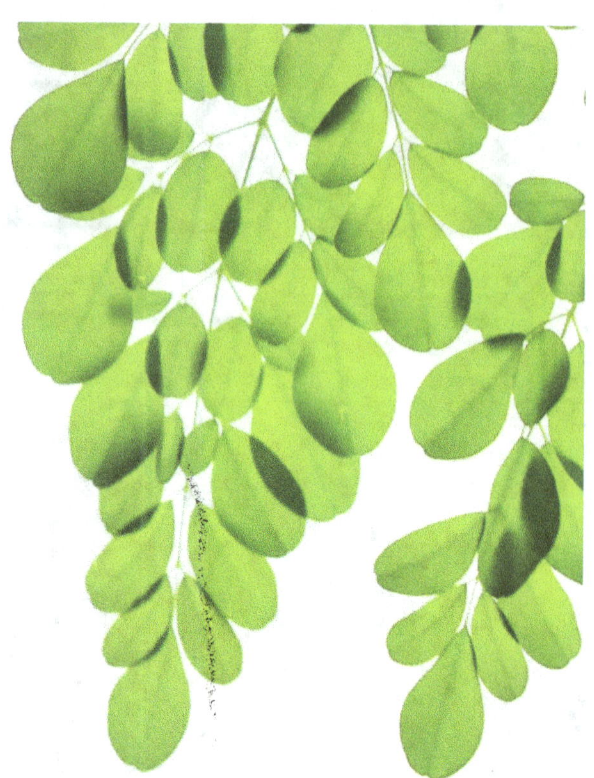

Ingredients

3-4 crabs
2 cups moringa leaves
½ cup freshly grated coconut
3 tsp cumin seeds
2 tsp feugreek seeds
2 tsp fennel seeds
3 tsp ground black pepper
¼ tsp turmeric powder
1 tbsp roasted chilli powder
1 tbsp coriander powder
1 tsp black mustard seeds
A golf ball-sized serving of tamarind pulp
3-4 large tomatoes, chopped
1 cup coconut milk
4 tbsp cooking oil
10-12 small red onions, sliced
¼ cup garlic and ginger paste
Handful of curry leaves
4-5 green chillies, finely chopped
Water as required
Salt to taste

Method

1. Clean the crabs—pull off the spongy grey gills and remove the guts. Chop each crab into two pieces.
2. In a dry frying pan over medium heat, toast the cumin seeds, coconut, and black pepper until the coconut is golden brown.
3. Place mixture in the blender and grind into a smooth paste.
4. Combine the tamarind and coconut milk in a small bowl. Mix until it forms a thick paste.
5. Heat oil in a large pot over high heat.
6. Add mustard seeds, fenugreek, and fennel seeds and lightly toast them.
7. Add onions, curry leaves, chillies, and garlic and ginger paste. Cook for a few minutes.
8. Add the chopped tomatoes and sauté for 10-15 minutes.
9. Add the turmeric powder, coriander powder, and chilli powder.
10. Mix well, then add the crabs. Cook for a few minutes.
11. Add the coconut paste. Toss and add a little water.
12. Cover the pot and let simmer for 15 minutes or until the crab is cooked.
13. Add the tamarind and milk paste.
14. Stir through and bring it to a boil
15. Remove from heat.
16. Mix in the moringa leaves. Season with sa' needed.
17. Serve hot with steamed white rice or *manto*.

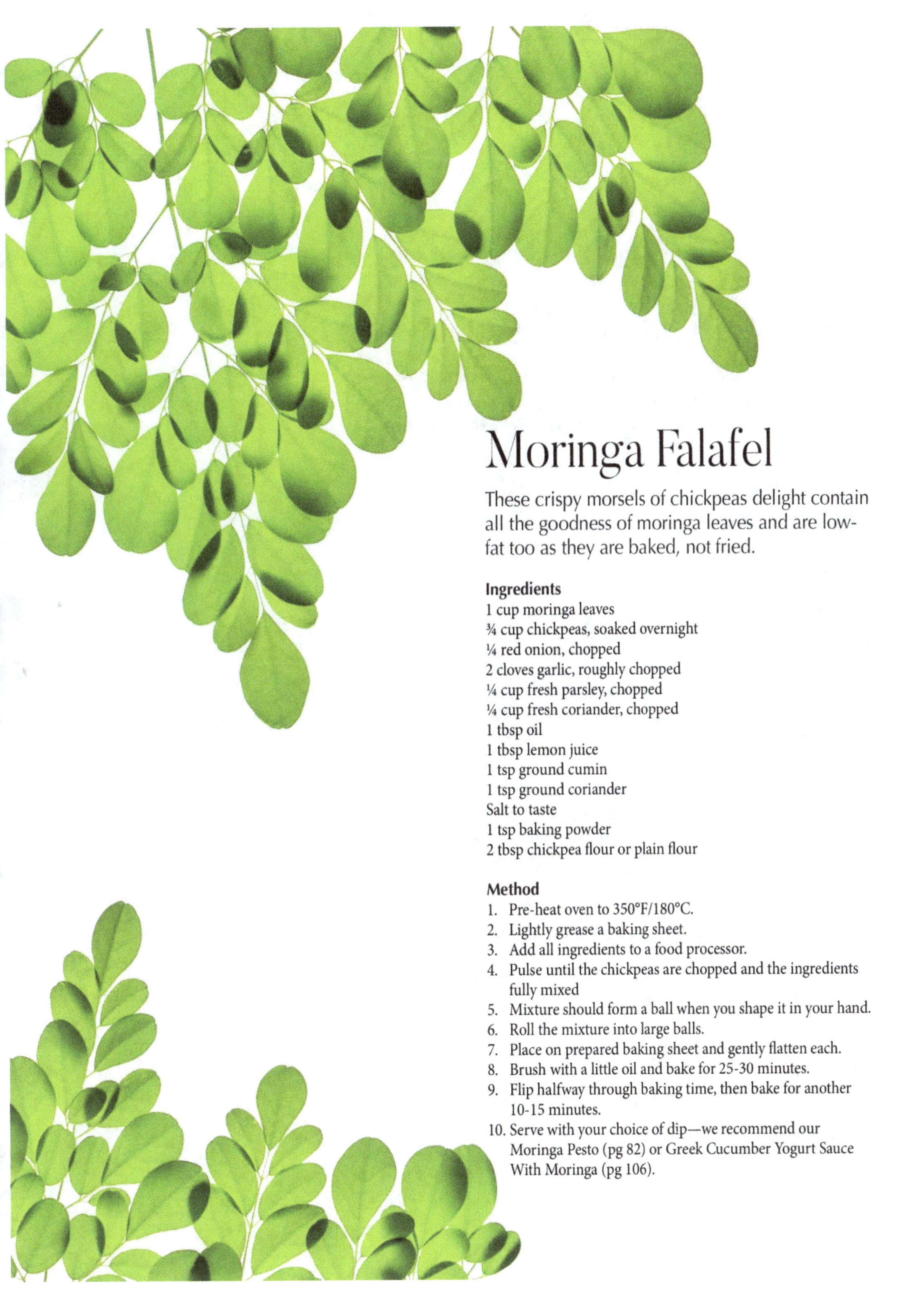

Moringa Falafel

These crispy morsels of chickpeas delight contain all the goodness of moringa leaves and are low-fat too as they are baked, not fried.

Ingredients

1 cup moringa leaves
¾ cup chickpeas, soaked overnight
¼ red onion, chopped
2 cloves garlic, roughly chopped
¼ cup fresh parsley, chopped
¼ cup fresh coriander, chopped
1 tbsp oil
1 tbsp lemon juice
1 tsp ground cumin
1 tsp ground coriander
Salt to taste
1 tsp baking powder
2 tbsp chickpea flour or plain flour

Method

1. Pre-heat oven to 350°F/180°C.
2. Lightly grease a baking sheet.
3. Add all ingredients to a food processor.
4. Pulse until the chickpeas are chopped and the ingredients fully mixed
5. Mixture should form a ball when you shape it in your hand.
6. Roll the mixture into large balls.
7. Place on prepared baking sheet and gently flatten each.
8. Brush with a little oil and bake for 25-30 minutes.
9. Flip halfway through baking time, then bake for another 10-15 minutes.
10. Serve with your choice of dip—we recommend our Moringa Pesto (pg 82) or Greek Cucumber Yogurt Sauce With Moringa (pg 106).

Moringa Leaves Paratha

Adding moringa leaves to everybody's favourite paratha makes it a protein-rich meal. Enjoy with dal or curry. Incidentally, this is one of Indian Prime Minister Narendra Modi's favourite dishes.

Ingredients
1 cup moringa leaves, chopped
2 cups atta flour
¼ cup *gram* flour (*besan*)
1 tsp green chillies, chopped
3 tbsp onion, chopped
1 tsp ginger, chopped
2 tbsp coriander seeds, pounded
2 tsp cumin seeds
Salt to taste
½ tsp turmeric
Water as required
A dash of oil
Ghee as required

Method
1. In a large bowl, mix the flour, chopped moringa leaves, besan, green chillies, onion, ginger, pounded coriander seeds, cumin, turmeric, and salt to taste.
2. Add water as required and knead it into a stiff dough.
3. Cover with some oil and set the dough aside to rest.
4. Divide the dough into small balls.
5. Flour your workspace generously and lightly flatten each ball of dough by pressing on it gently.
6. With a rolling pin, roll out each flattened ball and then brush with ghee.
7. Fold each piece into a 3-fold rectangle and brush on more ghee. Fold a gain into a square and roll it out again, maintaining the square shape.
8. Place a pan on medium heat.
9. Put the rolled out pieces of dough on the pan to fry, one at a time.
10. Flip twice to make sure it's cooked evenly on both sides.
11. Cook until small air pockets develop and the dough starts to darken in colour.
12. Drizzle more ghee on top and continue cooking until there are brown spots dotting each piece of the paratha.
13. Take it off the heat and serve hot. Pair with Moringa Flower Dal (pg 60).

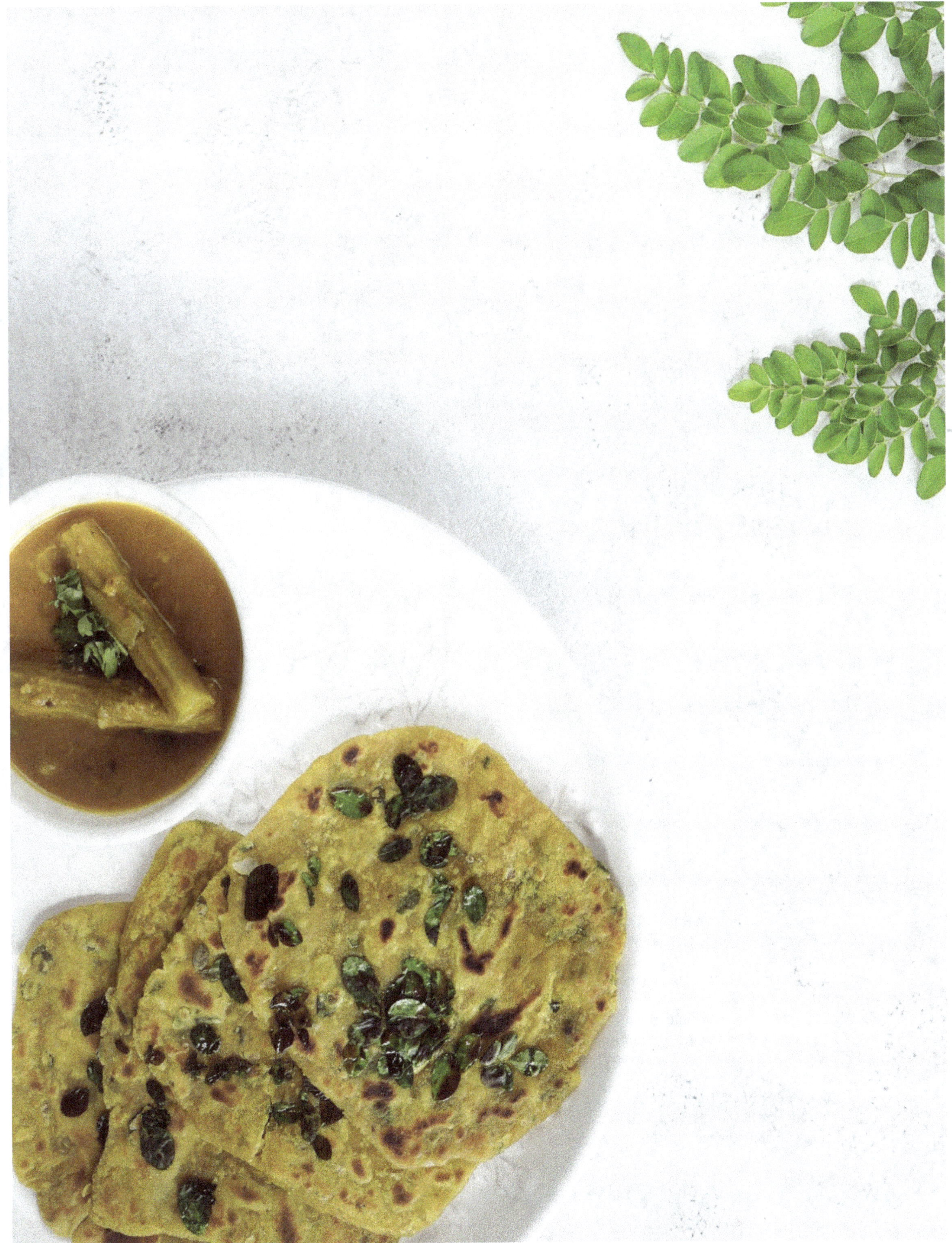

Moringa Pancakes

Everyone's favourite breakfast stack just got better with the addition of moringa leaves.

Ingredients
1 ½ cups all-purpose flour
3 ½ tsp baking powder
1 tbsp sugar
Salt to taste
1 ¼ cups milk
3 tbsp butter, melted
1 egg
1 cup moringa leaves

Method
1. Wash moringa leaves and boil for about two minutes.
2. Blend the leaves into a fine paste. Set aside.
3. Sift flour, baking powder, sugar, and salt into a large or mixing bowl.
4. Add milk, melted butter, egg, and the moringa leaves paste.
5. With a whisk, mix batter until smooth.
6. Heat a lightly-oiled pan over medium high heat.
7. Using a spoon or small ladle, scoop up the batter and pour onto the pan.
8. Cook for 2-3 minutes or until bubbles form.
9. Flip and cook the other side until browned.
10. Enjoy with honey or syrup of your choice.

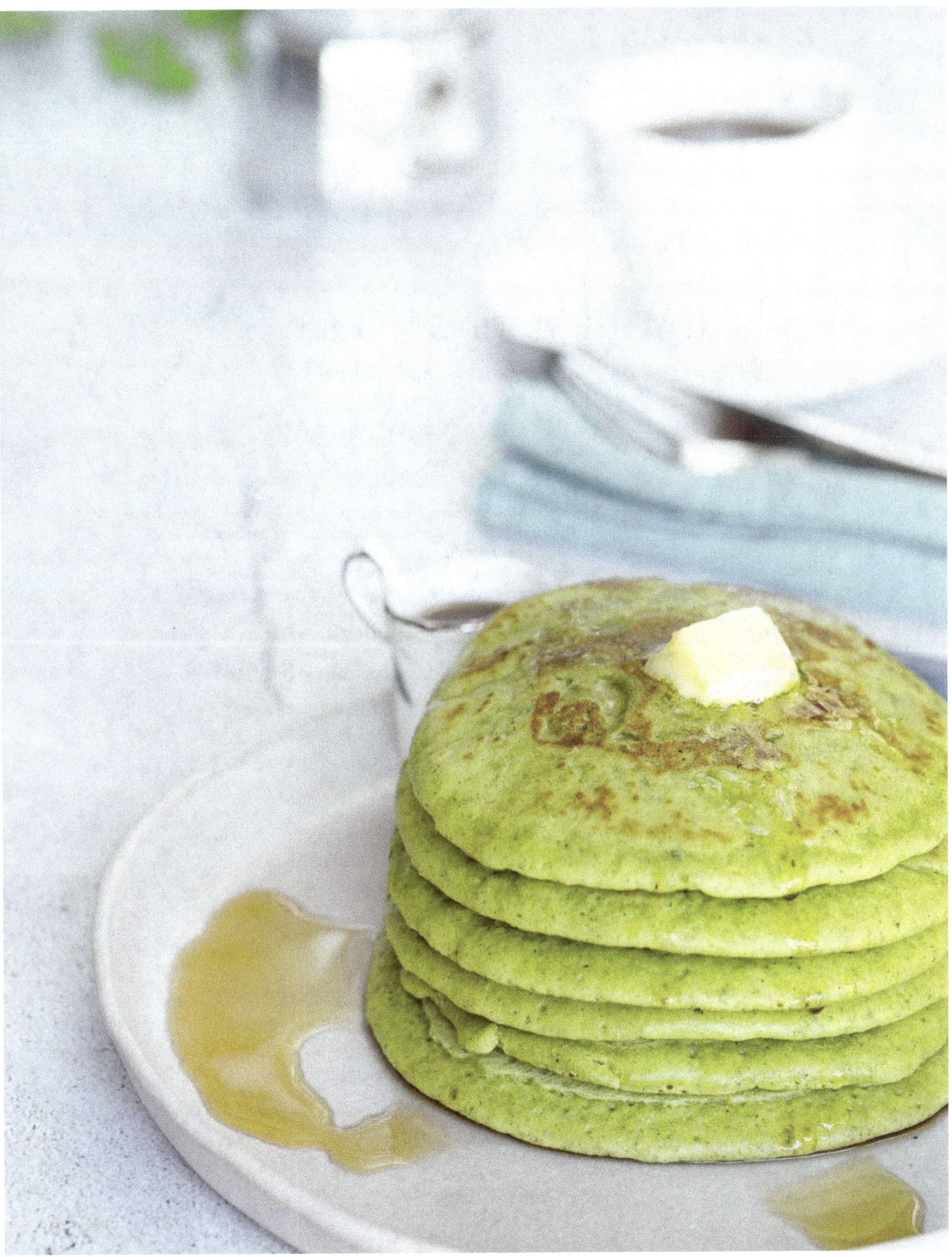

Spaghetti With Moringa Sauce

Give your usual pasta sauce a moringa twist by adding the fresh leaves.

Ingredients
Pasta of your choice
2 tbsp oil

For the sauce
3 tbsp oil
2 small onions
2 medium carrots
100gm green beans
1 medium tomato
3 cups moringa leaves
2 cups water

Method
1. Chop the carrots, onions, green beans, and tomato.
2. Pour oil into a pan.
3. Sauté the chopped vegetables and all the other ingredients for the sauce.
4. Once it's browned, add water and let simmer for a few minutes.
5. Remove pan from the heat.
6. Pour the sauce mixture into a blender and blitz into a puree.
7. Cook the pasta according to instructions on the packaging.
8. Sauté the cooked pasta in oil.
9. Add the sauce to the pan and toss to coat every piece or strand of the pasta evenly.
10. To serve, garnish with chopped tomatoes and a handful of fresh moringa leaves.

Moringa Pesto

Pesto is a rustic sauce made by grinding fresh basil leaves, pine nuts, garlic, salt, cheese, and olive oil. To make it more nutritious, use fresh moringa leaves in place of basil.

Ingredients
½ cup fresh moringa leaves
½ cup fresh basil leaves
Handful of fresh parsley
¼ cup toasted pine nuts
Zest of 1 lemon
1 clove garlic, peeled
½ cup grated parmesan (more if you like it really creamy)
Pinch of salt
Pinch of freshly ground black pepper
⅓ cup extra virgin olive oil

Method
1. Add all ingredients, except olive oil, to the bowl of a food processor or into a blender.
2. Process until everything is well-minced and blended.
3. Leave processor in the 'on' position and slowly drizzle in the olive oil until the mixture is well-blended.
4. Taste, and season as needed.
5. Cover tightly and refrigerate overnight.
6. Remove from refrigerator and allow to reach room temperature before using—toss into your choice of pasta, spread it onto a sandwich, or add to fried or poached eggs for breakfast.

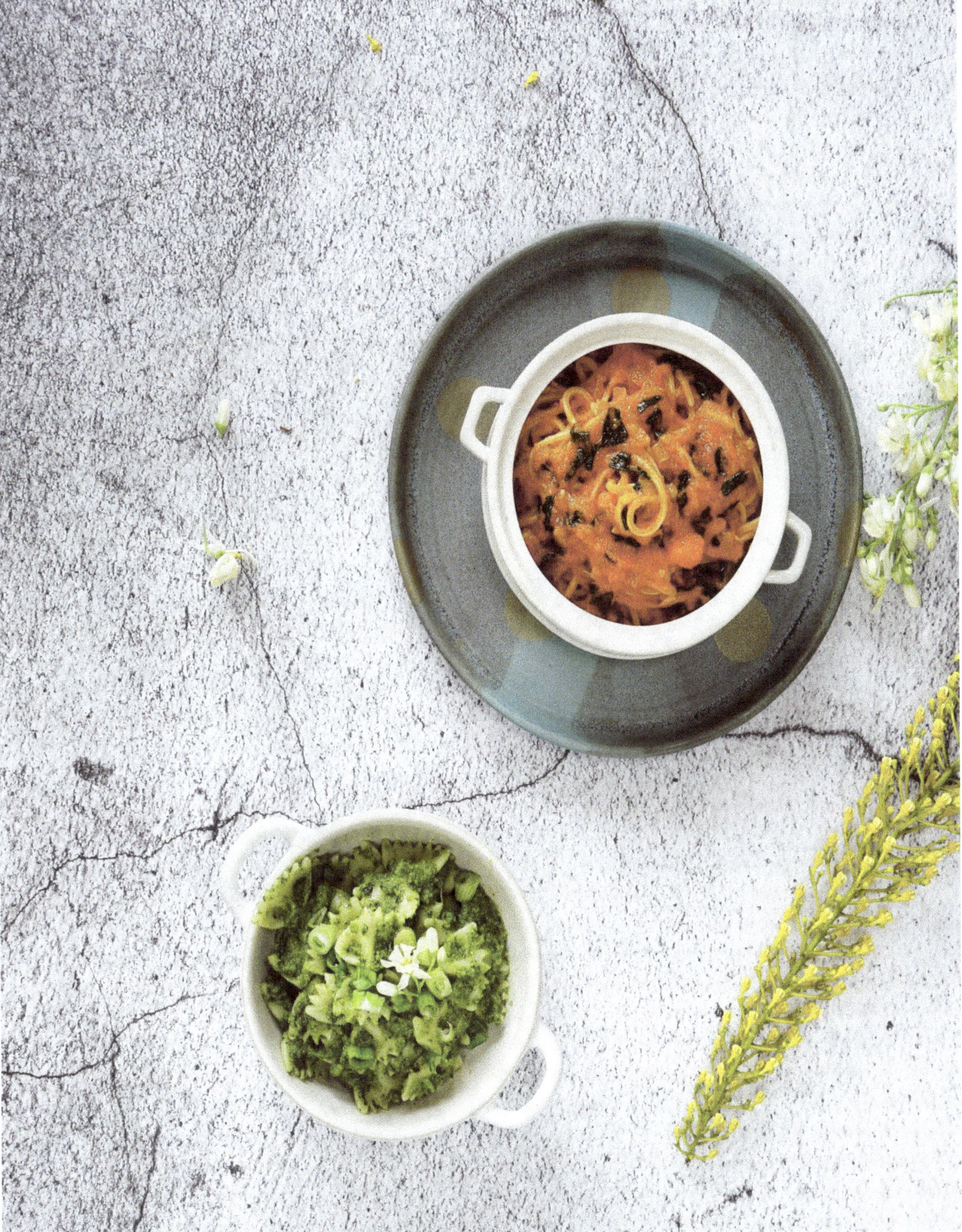

Stir-Fried Shrimps With Moringa Leaves

This simple stir-fry is one of the easiest, quickest, and most nutritious dishes you can put on the dinner table!

Ingredients
½ cup moringa leaves
1 head of bok choy
200gm shrimps
3 tbsp soy sauce
2 tbsp fresh ginger
¼ tsp chilli paste
4 pieces spring onions
3 garlic cloves
3 tbsp oil
10-15 shiitake mushrooms
2 red bell peppers

Method
1. Peel and devein shrimps.
2. Add finely chopped ginger, soy sauce, chopped garlic, and onions.
3. Toss well and marinate for 30 minutes.
4. Heat 2 tbsp oil in a wok.
5. Drain shrimps, while preserving the marinade.
6. Add shrimps to the wok and stir-fry for 2 minutes.
7. Remove shrimp from wok and set aside.
8. Bring water to boil and add moringa leaves, and cook for 2 minutes
9. Add remaining oil to wok.
10. Add shitake mushrooms and cook for 2 minutes.
11. Add moringa leaves, chopped bok choy, and red bell peppers.
12. Cook for an additional 5 minutes.
13. Add shrimps, mix well, and simmer for 2 more minutes.
14. Serve hot with steamed rice.

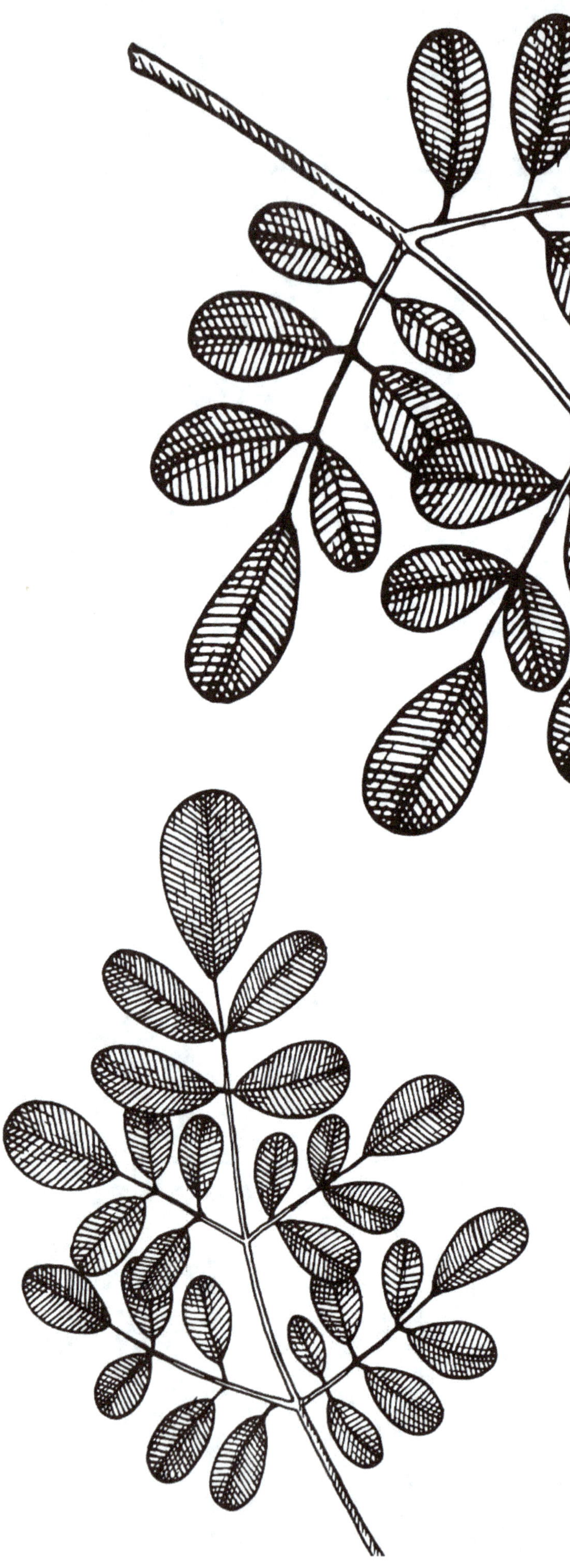

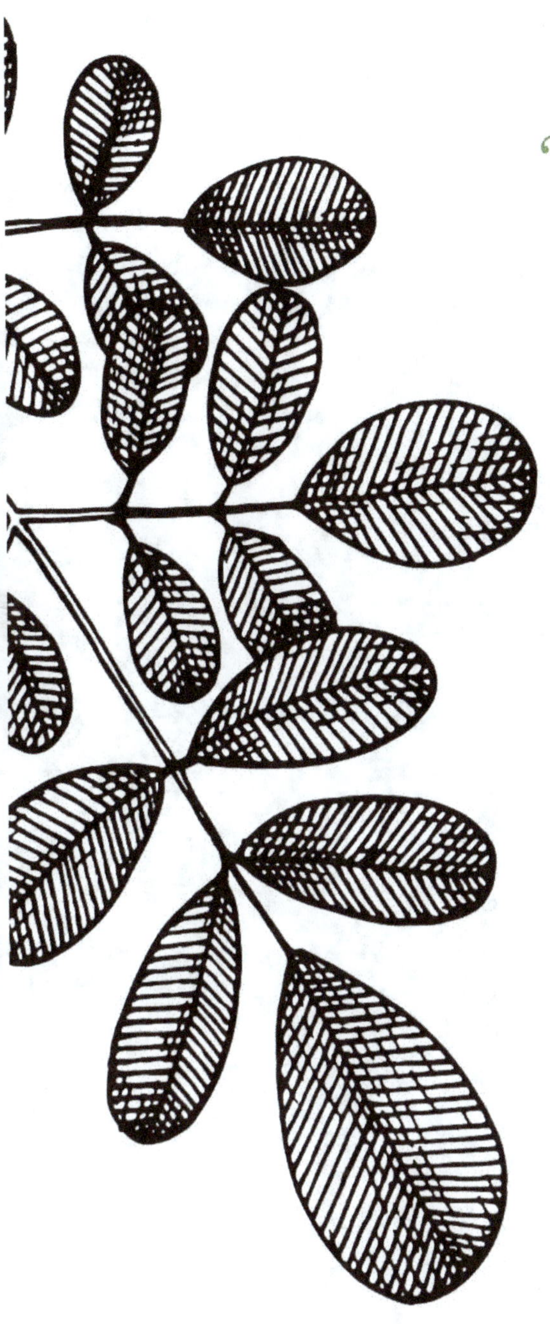

Myanmarese Moringa Leaf Soup

In Myanmarese cuisine, soups typically accompany meals featuring both rice and noodles. The soups are usually lightly flavoured and paired accordingly to balance contrasting flavours. This simple soup can be served with almost all meals.

Ingredients
1 medium onion, chopped
2-3 cloves of garlic, chopped
1/2 inch ginger, chopped
4 cups water
3 cups moringa leaves
Salt and pepper to taste

Method
1. Place onion, garlic, and ginger into a pot with the water.
2. Bring to a boil.
3. Add moringa leaves and cook until wilted.
4. Taste, then season with salt and pepper as needed.
5. Serve as part of a meal

Note:
The leaves must be added last and should be cooked only for a few minutes.

Moringa Rainbow Salad

An easy salad that is vibrant, colourful and packed with flavoured and nutrients.

Ingredients

For the salad
1-2 cups moringa leaves
1-2 sweet peppers (red, yellow or green or a combination)
½ cup tomatoes, chopped
1 cucumber, chopped

For the dressing
½ cup olive oil
1 tbsp honey
2 tbsp balsamic vinegar
2-3 cloves garlic, chopped
Few sprigs of fresh thyme (or ¼ tsp dried thyme) (optional)
Salt and pepper to taste

Method
1. Place all the salad ingredients into a bowl.
2. In a separate bowl, mix the dressing ingredients.
3. Just before serving, drizzle the dressing onto the ingredients and toss.
4. Add chopped nuts of your choice. (optional)
5. Serve immediately.

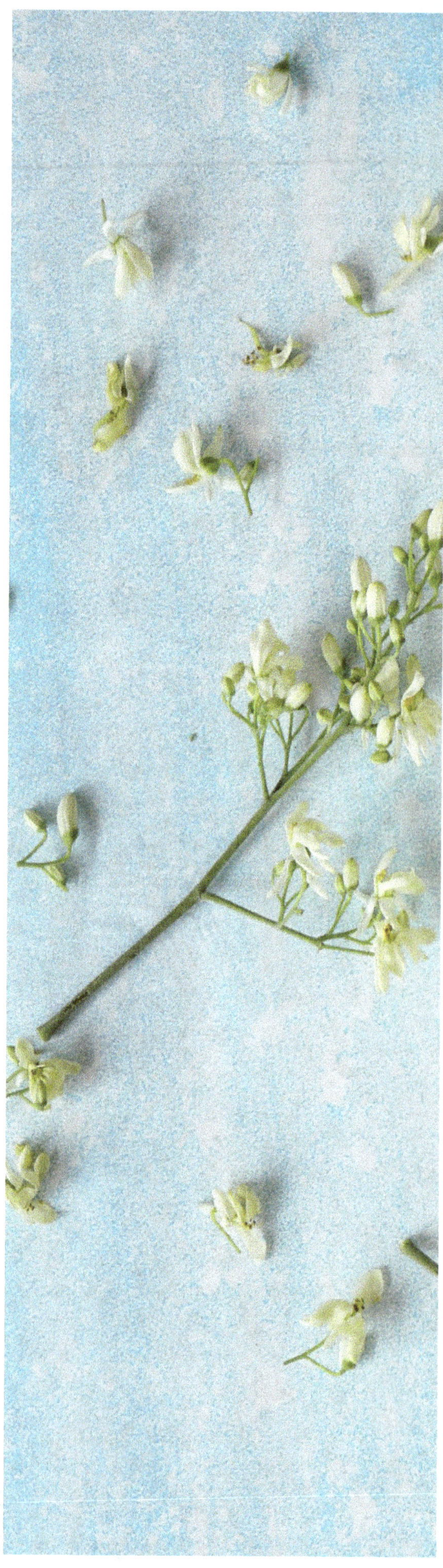

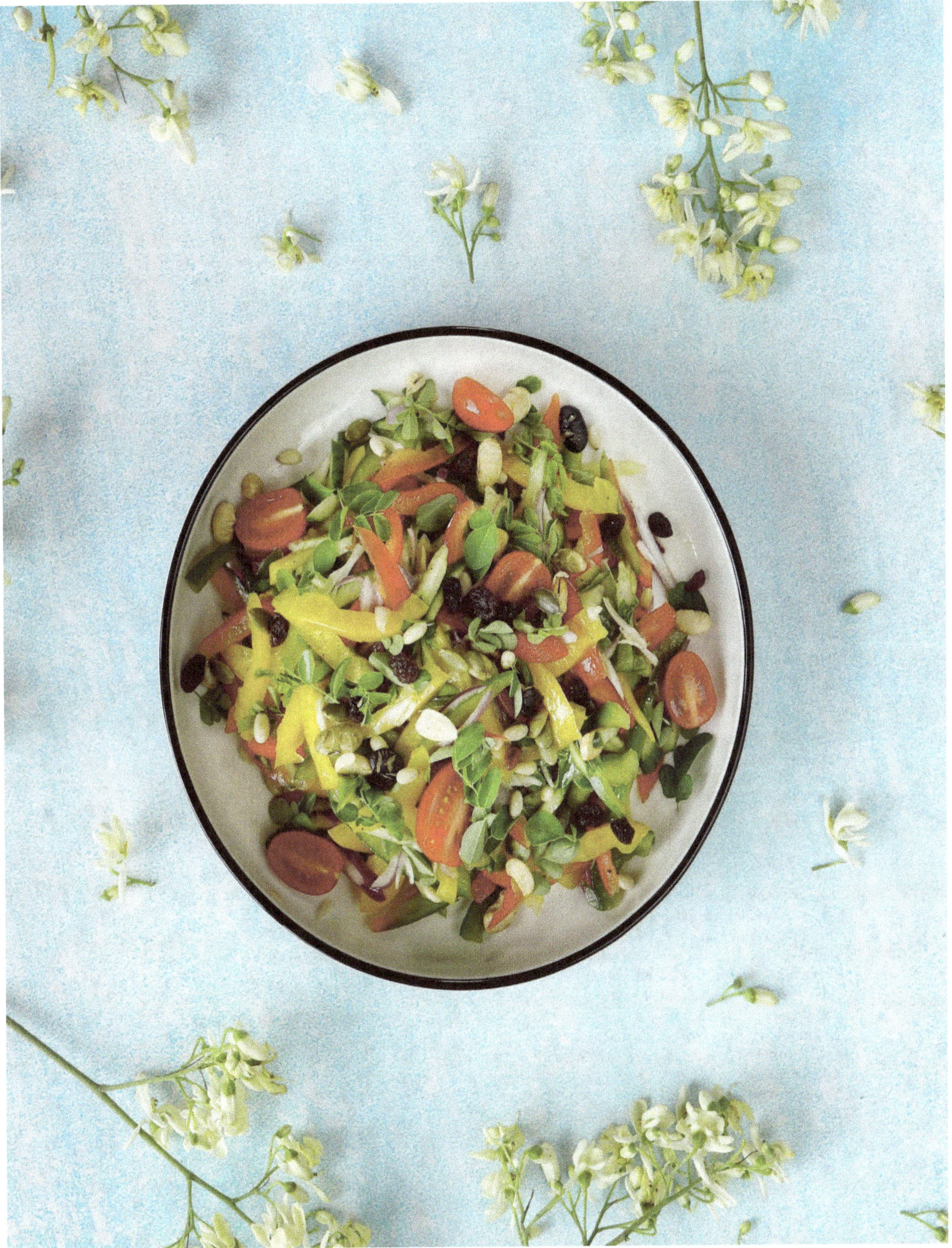

Moringa Leaves Rice

A wonderful mix of greens, spices, and of course moringa takes this basmati rice dish to another level!

Ingredients
2 tbsp oil
1 bay leaf
2 cloves
1-inch cinnamon stick
1 tsp cumin seeds
1 medium onion, finely chopped
1 cup moringa leaves
½ cup green peas
2 cups cooked basmati rice
½ tsp turmeric powder
Salt to taste

For grinding
¼ cup coriander leaves
¼ cup mint leaves
3-4 green chillies
2 cloves garlic
1-2 inch ginger
2-3 tbsp water

Method
1. Place all the ingredients for grinding into a blender or food processor and blitz into a smooth paste.
2. Heat 2 tbsp oil in a pan.
3. Add whole spices, bayleaf, cloves, cinnamon, and cumin seeds. Let them splutter for a few seconds.
4. Add the onions and sauté until light brown.
5. Add the ground ingredients.
6. Add moringa leaves, green peas, turmeric, and salt.
7. Cook for another 2-3 minutes until the leaves wilt.
8. Add the cooked rice.
9. Mix well, then turn off the gas.
10. Serve hot with your favourite side dishes. (Try it with our Chicken with Moringa Leaves, pg 96)

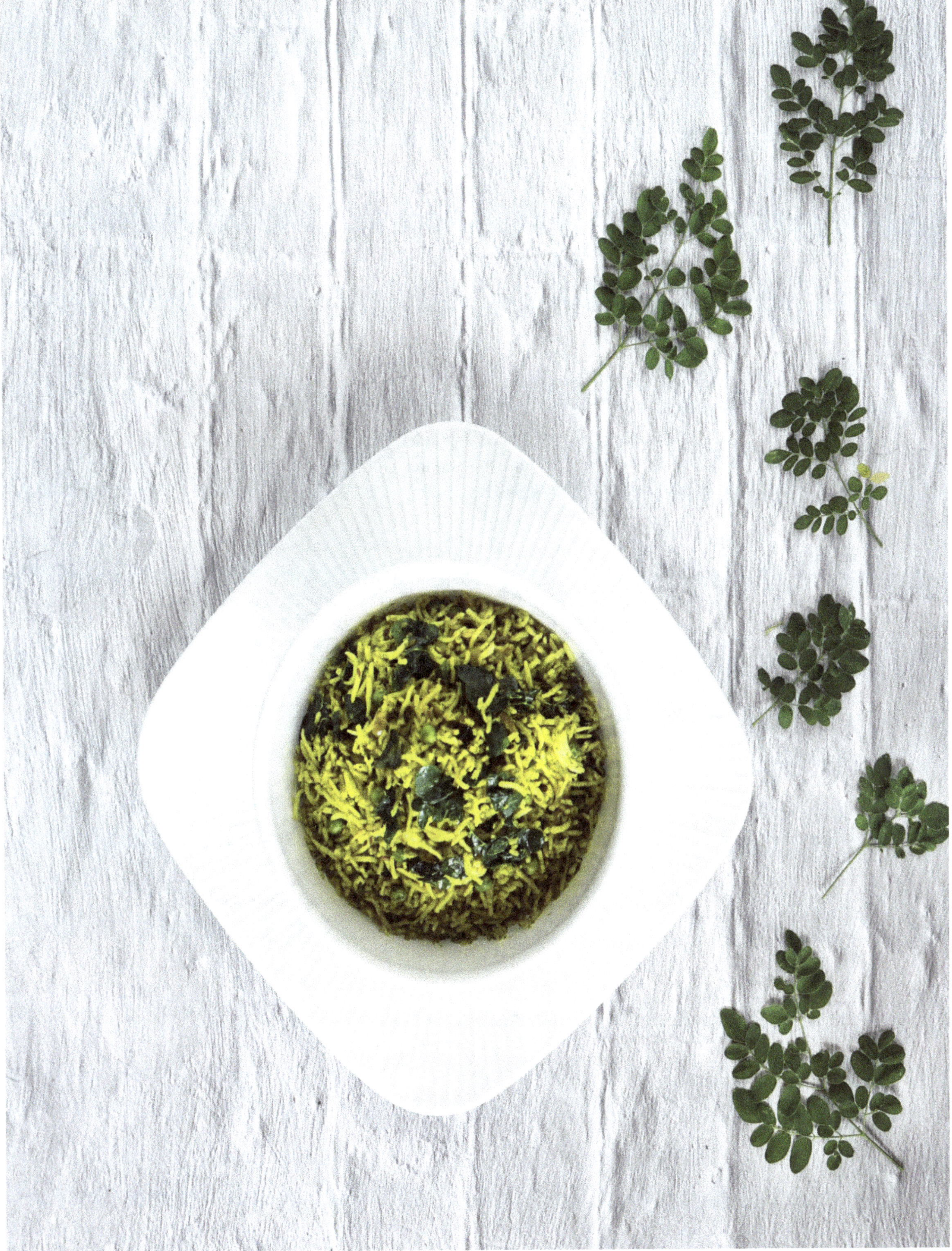

Nasi Lemak Moringa

Nasi lemak is the de facto national dish of Malaysia, a colourful platter that's rich in flavours and textures. Take it a step further—add fresh moringa leaves into the coconut milk rice for a nutritious treat!

Ingredients
1 cup rice
1-2 screw pine leaves (*daun pandan*)
1 ½ cups coconut milk
½ cup moringa leaves

(Tamarind juice)
½ cup water
Tamarind pulp (size of half a ping pong ball)

(Sambal)
½ red onion
1 clove garlic
2 shallots
5-6 dried chillies
Salt to taste
½ tbsp sugar

For garnishing/as condiments
Eggs your way
½ cup anchovies
½ cup roasted peanuts
½ cucumber, sliced

Two ways to infuse moringa into this dish:
a) Blend a handful of fresh moringa leaves in the coconut milk and cook the rice with it.
b) Chop up the moringa leaves. Cook the rice in coconut milk. When it's almost ready, add the leaves into the rice and toss it well.

Method
1. Rinse rice and drain.
2. Add coconut milk, a pinch of salt, and screw pine leaves.
3. Cook in rice cooker until done.
4. Fry the anchovies in a little oil until crispy. Set aside.

(For the *sambal*)
1. Soak the tamarind pulp in water for 15 minutes.
2. Squeeze the tamarind to extract its flavour. Set aside.
3. Pound the shallots, onions, garlic, and dried chillies into a thick paste.
4. Heat some oil in a pan.
5. Fry until the paste is fragrant.
6. Add the tamarind juice, salt, and sugar.
7. Simmer on low heat until the *sambal* thickens.
8. To serve, place a bowlful of rice in the middle of the serving plate. Top with the *sambal*. Place the egg, cucumber slices, roasted peanuts, and crispy anchovies around the rice.

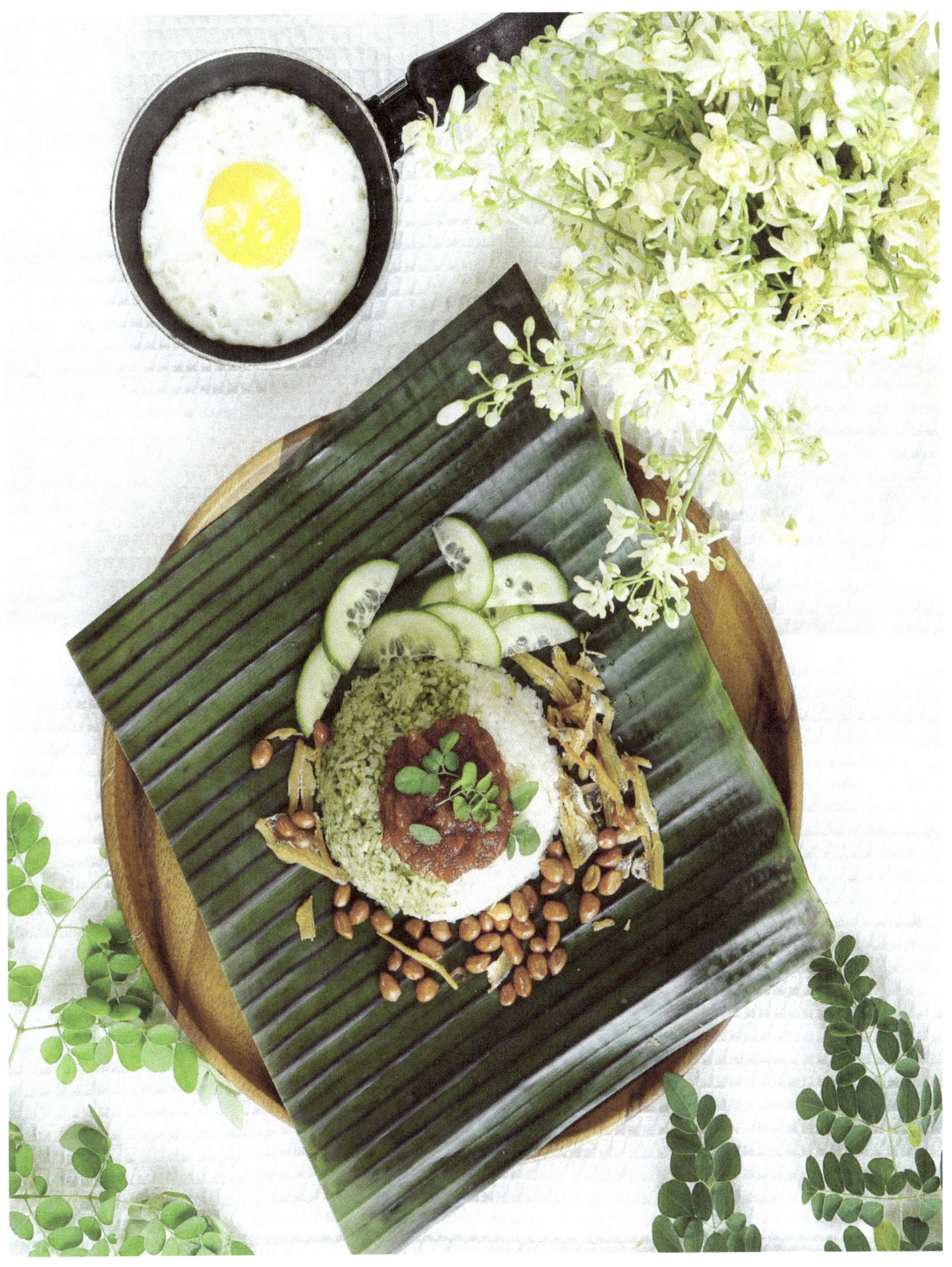

Khauk Swe (Burmese-Style Curry Noodles)

This is a popular dish throughout Myanmar and a family favourite when I was growing up. It is similar to the *khao soi* of northern Thailand and bears Indian-Muslim influence, as indicated by the use of *garam masala*. The rich curry chicken broth gets a tangy, appetising lift when you add a squeeze of fresh lime juice.

Ingredients
500g chicken breast fillet
1 tsp fish sauce
Salt to taste
3 tbsp cooking oil
1 tsp sweet paprika
½ tsp ground cumin
1 tsp garam masala
2 onions, peeled and chopped
3 cloves of garlic, peeled and chopped
1-inch knob of ginger, peeled and chopped
One cup chicken stock
3 tbsp roasted chickpea flour
1 cup thick coconut milk
12 shallots, peeled and pureed
220gm fresh yellow noodles, blanched

For garnishing
3 hard-boiled eggs, peeled and sliced
2 onions, peeled and finely sliced, then soaked in water and squeezed
¼ cup spring onions, chopped
¼ cup coriander leaves, chopped
1¼ cup moringa leaves, chopped
1 tbsp chili flakes
2-3 fresh limes, cut into wedges

Method
1. Marinate the chicken with the fish sauce and some salt. Set aside for 10 minutes.
2. Heat oil in saucepan, add onion garlic and ginger turmeric, paprika, cumin, garam masala, and stir-fry for a few minutes.
3. Add the chicken and cook for a few minutes.
4. Add the chicken stock and bring to a boil.
5. Mix the chickpea flour with a small amount of water. Stir into the simmering stock.
6. Add the coconut milk and allow stock to simmer.
7. Add the shallots and let cook for a few minutes.
8. Divide the noodles among individual serving bowls and ladle the broth over.
9. Top with hard-boiled egg, sliced onions, spring onions, coriander, chilli flakes, and lime wedges.
10. Garnish with some moringa leaves just before serving.

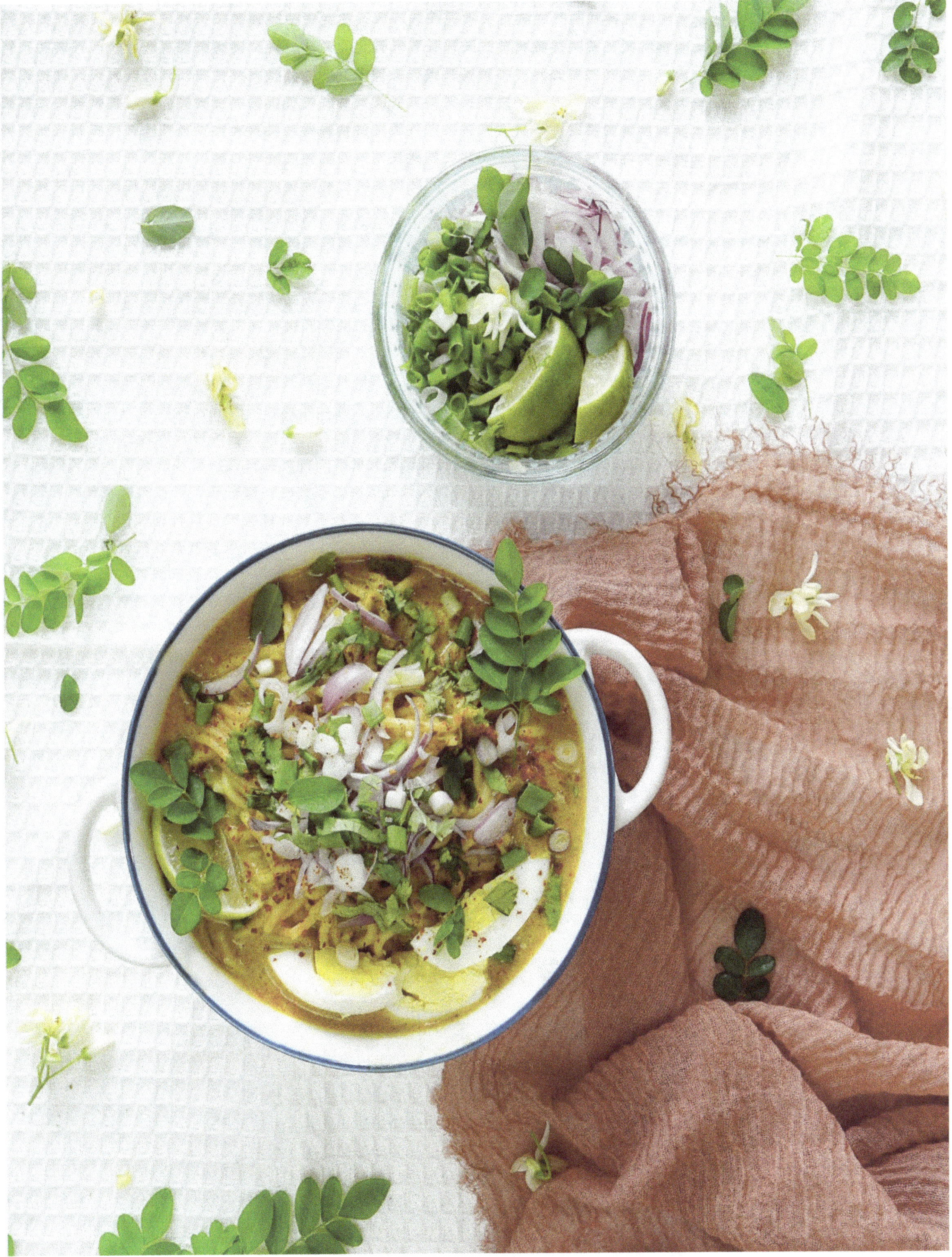

Moringa Leaves Stir-Fried With Grated Coconut

Mildly spicy with a nutty aroma, this delicious and nutritious dish brings out the best of freshly grated coconut and moringa leaves.

Ingredients
6 cups moringa leaves
¼ tsp turmeric powder
1 ¼ cup grated coconut
Salt to taste
1 tbsp oil
½ tsp mustard seeds
¼ cup shallots, finely chopped
1 tbsp crushed dried chillies
1 stalk curry leaves

Method
1. Place moringa leaves, grated coconut, turmeric powder, and salt in a mixing bowl. Combine well.
2. Heat oil in a pan.
3. Splutter the mustard seeds, then add the chopped shallots.
4. When the shallots turn translucent, add the crushed chillies and curry leaves,
5. Sauté for a few minutes over medium heat.
6. Add the moringa leaves mixture and toss to mix everything together.
7. Close the lid and cook for a few minutes.
8. Open lid, stir well and sauté for a few more minutes.
9. Add salt to taste.
10. Serve hot with rice and curry.

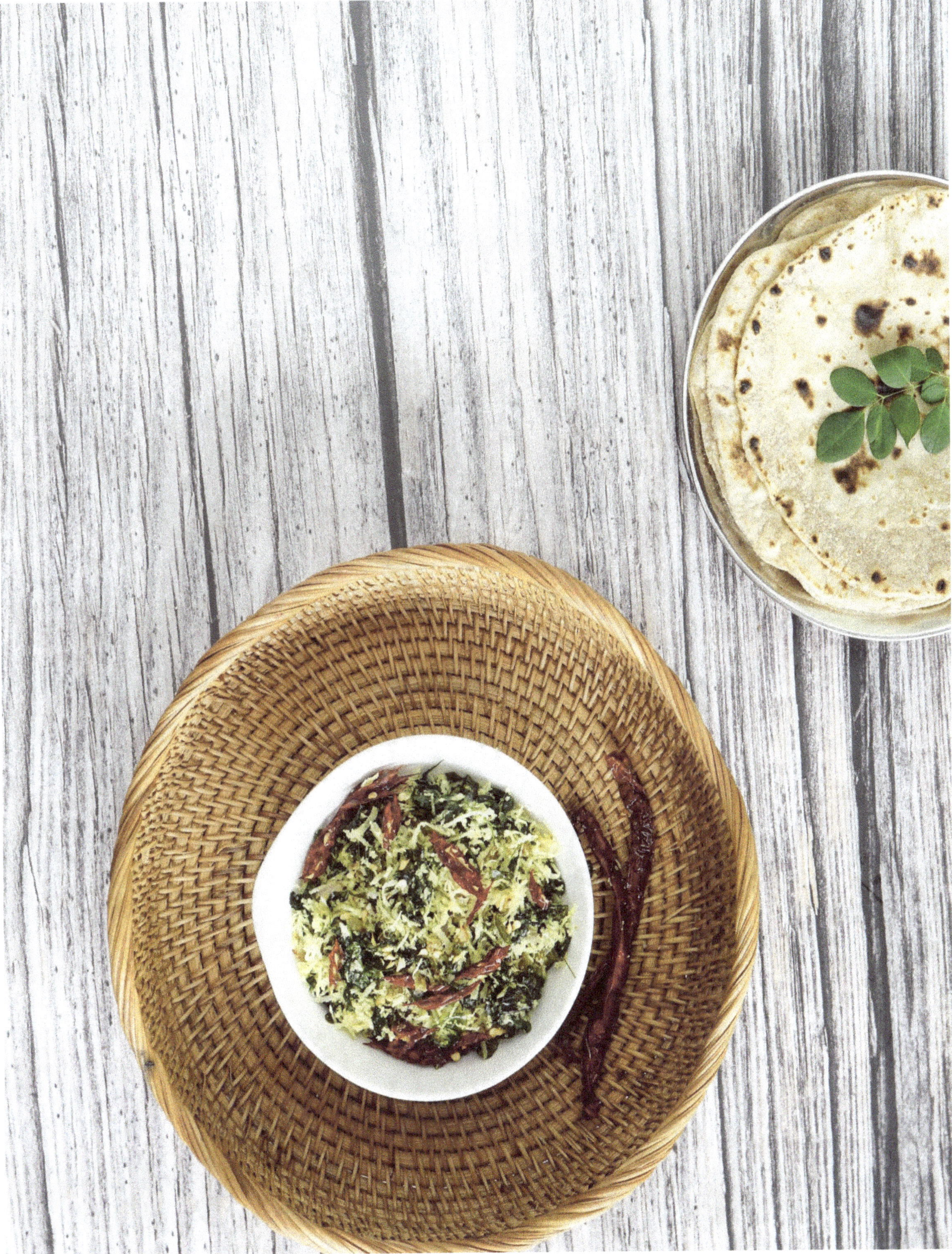

Chicken With Moringa Leaves

We promise this is finger-licking delicious! Try this and it could be your favourite way to enjoy moringa.

Ingredients
500g chicken drumsticks (or any other parts of a chicken)
2 large onions, diced
1-2 tomatoes, pureed
1 ½ cups moringa leaves
A handful of curry leaves
1 tsp ginger-garlic paste
1 tsp red chilli powder
1 tsp coriander powder
1 tsp mustard seeds
1 tbsp oil
Salt to taste

Method
1. Heat oil in a pan.
2. Add mustard seeds and curry leaves.
3. When the seeds splutter, add sliced onions.
4. Fry until they turn golden brown.
5. Add the dry spices.
6. Sauté for two minutes.
7. Add tomato puree and cook 2-3 minutes.
8. Add the chicken and cook until tender.
9. Add moringa leaves.
10. Mix well.
11. Serve hot with bread, roti or rice .

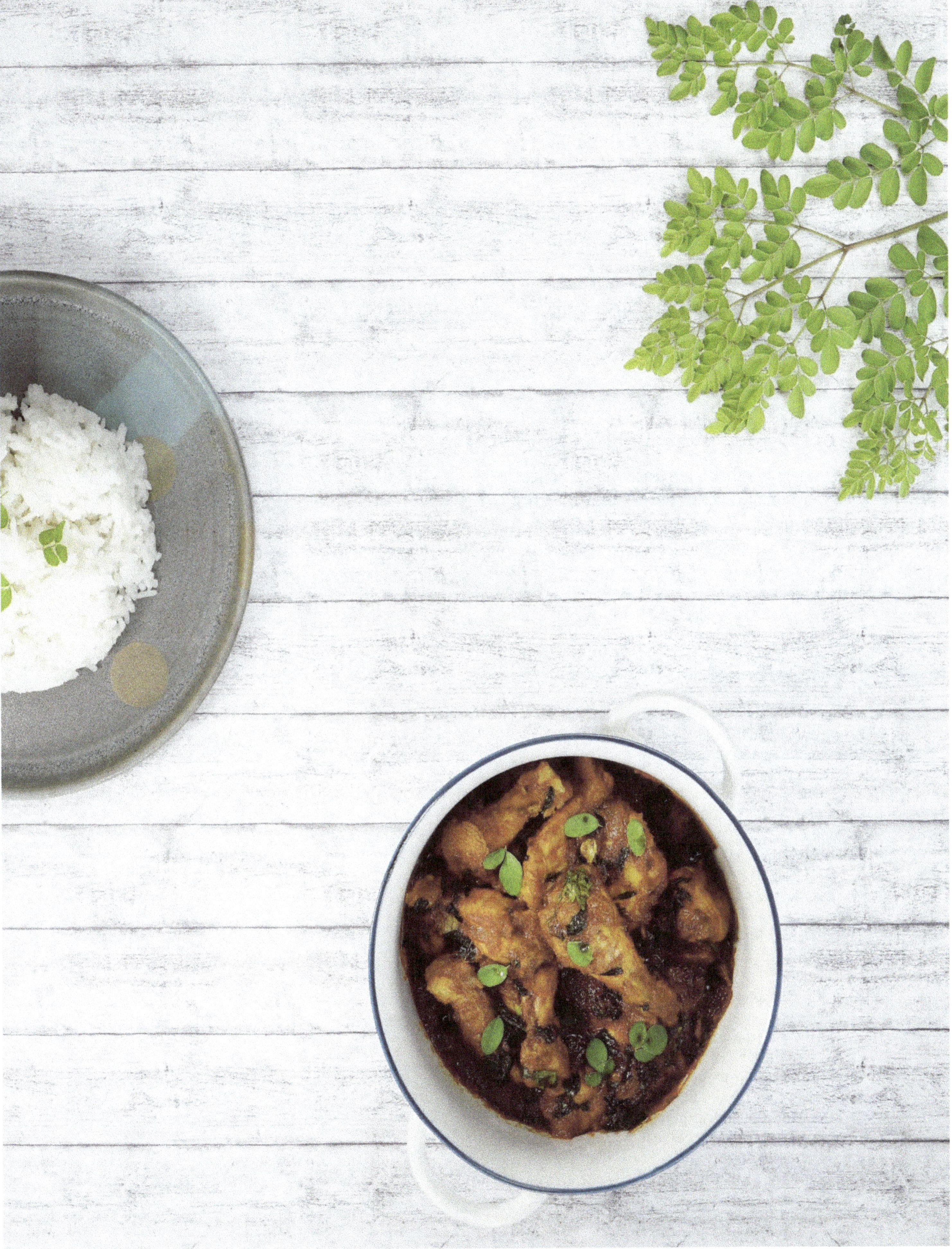

Prawns Moringa Vada

The perfect afternoon tea treat and TV snack!
We recommend pairing these crispy delights
with a mug of Moringa Flower Masala Milk.

Ingredients

200gm *channa dal* soaked for a few hours
200gm fresh moringa leaves
200gm fresh prawns, shelled and cleaned
1 tsp chopped ginger and garlic
1 onion, chopped
2-3 green chillies, chopped
½ tsp garam masala
½ tsp ground cumin
½ tsp chilli powder or to taste
Salt and pepper to taste

Method

1. Set aside a handful of the soaked *channa dal*.
2. Add remaining *channa dal* and moringa leaves in a mixer
   and grind to a paste.
3. Add prawns and blitz a few times.
4. Transfer to a bowl.
5. Add chopped onions, chopped ginger and garlic, and green
   chillies.
6. Add cumin powder, chilli powder, garam masala, and salt
   and pepper.
7. Mix well and let rest for a few minutes. Add the handful of
   channa dal that was set aside earlier to the mixture.
8. With a tablespoon or your hands, scoop a small amount of
   the mixture onto your palms and shape into discs. Flatten slightly.
9. Fry in hot oil on medium heat until crisp.
10. Serve with dip or chutney of your choice.

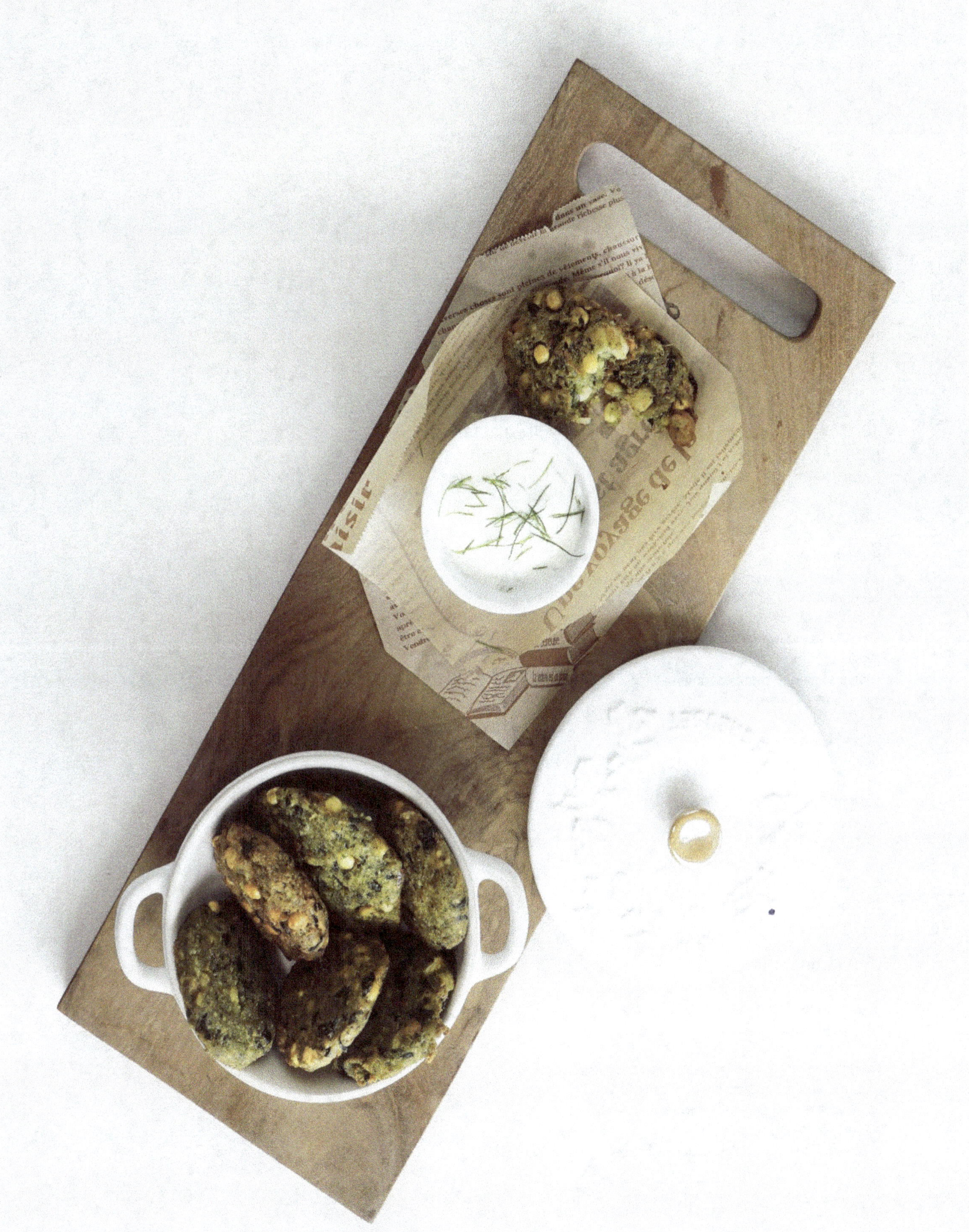

Moroccan-Style Stuffed Peppers With Moringa

The savoury flavours of the stuffing pair well with the
natural sweetness of the bell peppers. You can also
bake them in an airfryer.

Ingredients
3 bell peppers, halved
150gm couscous
300ml vegetable stock
400g chickpeas, washed and cooked
100gm crumbled
100gm tomatoes, chopped roughly
A few olives, chopped
Juice of ½ lemon
3 tbsp olive oil
2 cups moringa leaves

Method
1. Pre-heat oven to 400°F/200°C.
2. Cut peppers into half and remove the seeds.
3. Place peppers on a baking tray, cut side up.
4. Roast in the oven for 20-25 minutes
5. Place couscous in a bowl and pour the hot stock over.
6. Cover and let stand 5-10 minutes.
7. Use a fork to fluff the couscous.
8. Stir in the chickpeas, feta, tomatoes, olives, lemon juice, and olive oil.
9. Add the moringa leaves.
10. Season with salt and pepper.
11. Take the peppers out of the oven and fill them with the couscous mixture.
12. Return the peppers to the oven and roast for a further 10-15 minutes.
13. Serve with extra feta cheese over the top.

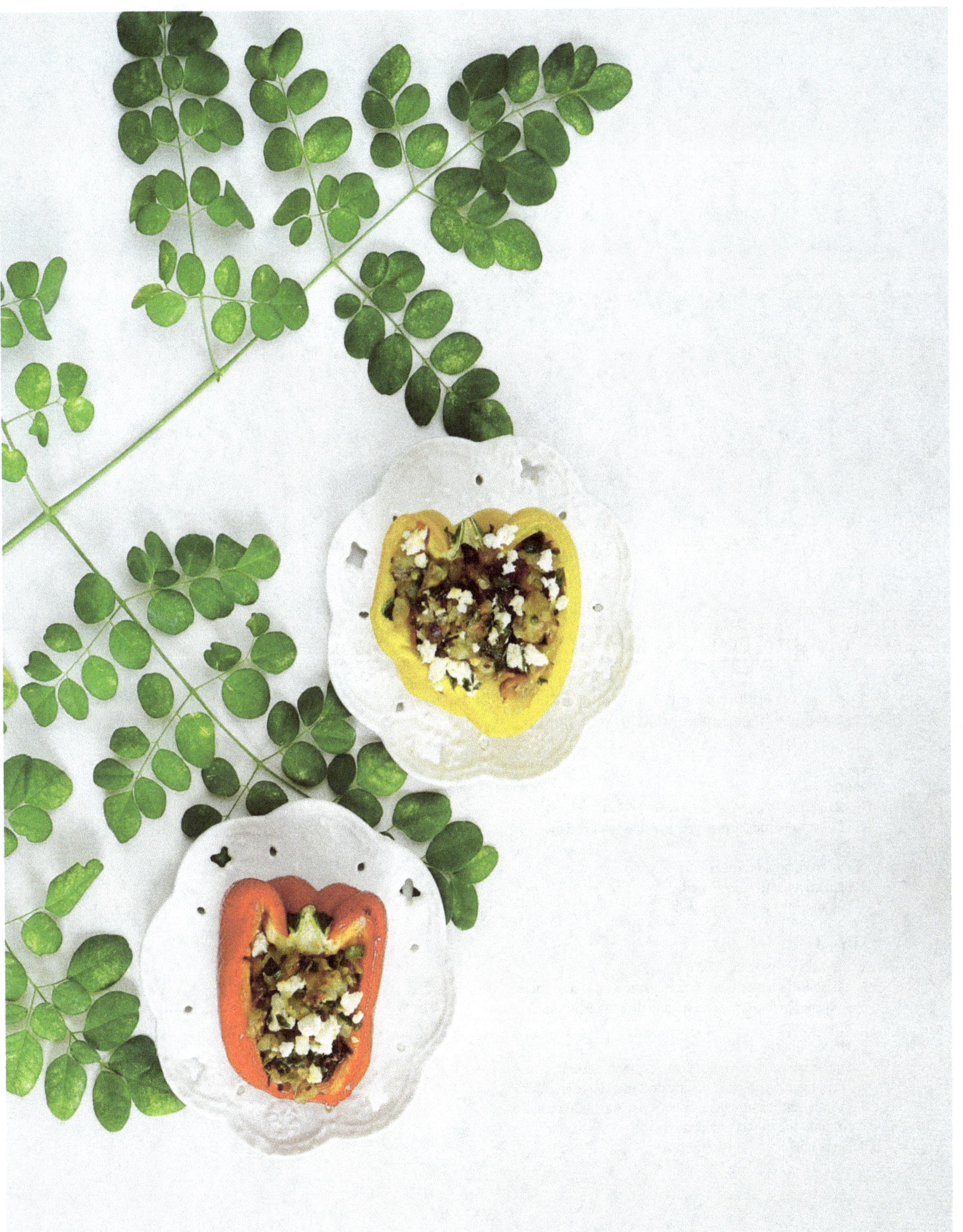

Moringa-Stuffed Mushrooms

Great as an appetiser or tea time snack, these are easy to make and boast of a robust, umami flavour in a single bite.

Ingredients
Cooking spray
10-12 medium mushrooms, remove the stem and dice.
1 tbsp oil
¼ cup fresh bread crumbs
100gm cream cheese, softened
¾ cup moringa leaves, chopped

Method
1. Pre-heat oven to 400°F/200°C.
2. Combine bread crumbs, onion, garlic, and cream cheese.
3. Add chopped moringa leaves and diced mushroom stems.
4. Season with salt and pepper.
5. Hollow out the mushrooms.
6. Spoon the combined mixture into the mushrooms.
7. Place them on an oiled baking dish in a single layer.
8. Drizzle a little more oil over and bake for 15-20 minutes
   (or until the tops are golden brown).
9. Serve hot.

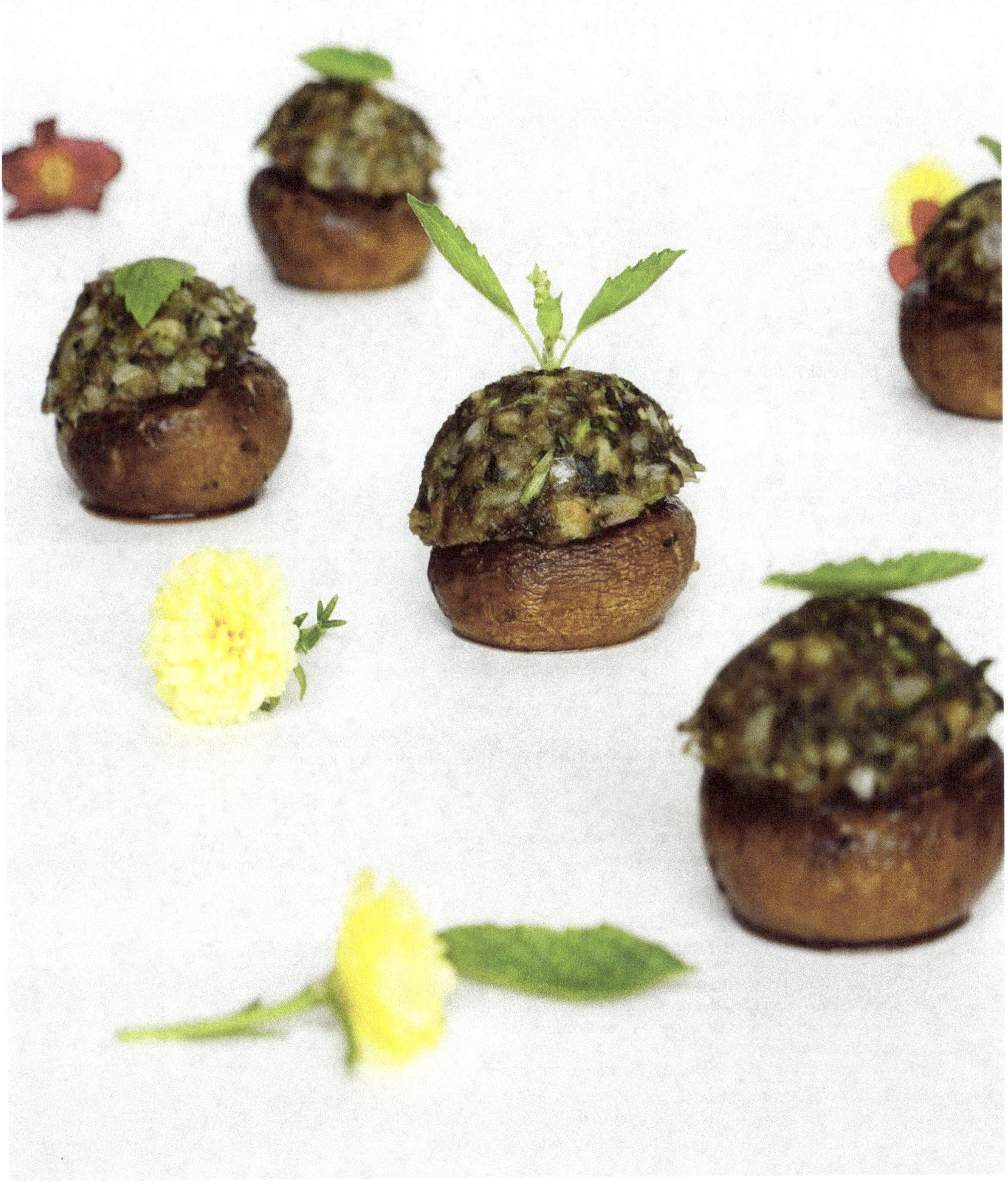

Moringa Dumpling Fritters (Muthias)

This Gujarati dish earned its moniker from the hand-gripping action involved in its making. *Muthias* can be steamed or fried, and comes in many varieties. I like it made from wheat flour and moringa leaves.

Ingredients
1 big bowl moringa leaves
1 ½ cup whole wheat flour
Oil for deep-frying

For the spice mix
½ tsp sesame seeds
¼ tsp carom seeds
1 tsp green chilli and ginger paste
½ tsp garlic paste
1 small onion, chopped
1 tsp turmeric powder
1 tsp cumin powder
1 tsp coriander powder
½ tsp fennel seeds
2-3 tbsp yogurt
½ tsp sugar
Pinch of baking powder
Pinch of *asefoetida*
2-3 tbsp oil
Salt to taste

Method
1. In a big bowl, mix the flour and the moringa leaves.
2. Add all the spices.
3. Mix thoroughly by hand.
4. Scoop a bit of the mixture onto your palms and mould it into a cylindrical shape.
5. Place the *muthias* in a steamer.
6. Steam for 10-15 minutes.
7. Remove *muthias* from the steamer and let cool.
8. For a different texture, you can also deep fry the *muthias* after steaming.
9. Enjoy them by dipping into sesame oil or peanut oil.

Method II
Here's another way to make *muthias*:
1. After mixing the batter, roll into a log.
2. Slice into round discs of about 2cm in thickness.
3. In a heavy bottom pan, add 2-3 tbsp oil. Sauté mustard seeds, sesame seeds, 2-3 whole red chillies, and a pinch of *asafoetida*.
4. Once the seeds begin to splutter, add the sliced dumplings and cook until they reach the desired crispiness.
5. Garnish with chopped coriander and add a squeeze of fresh lemon juice.

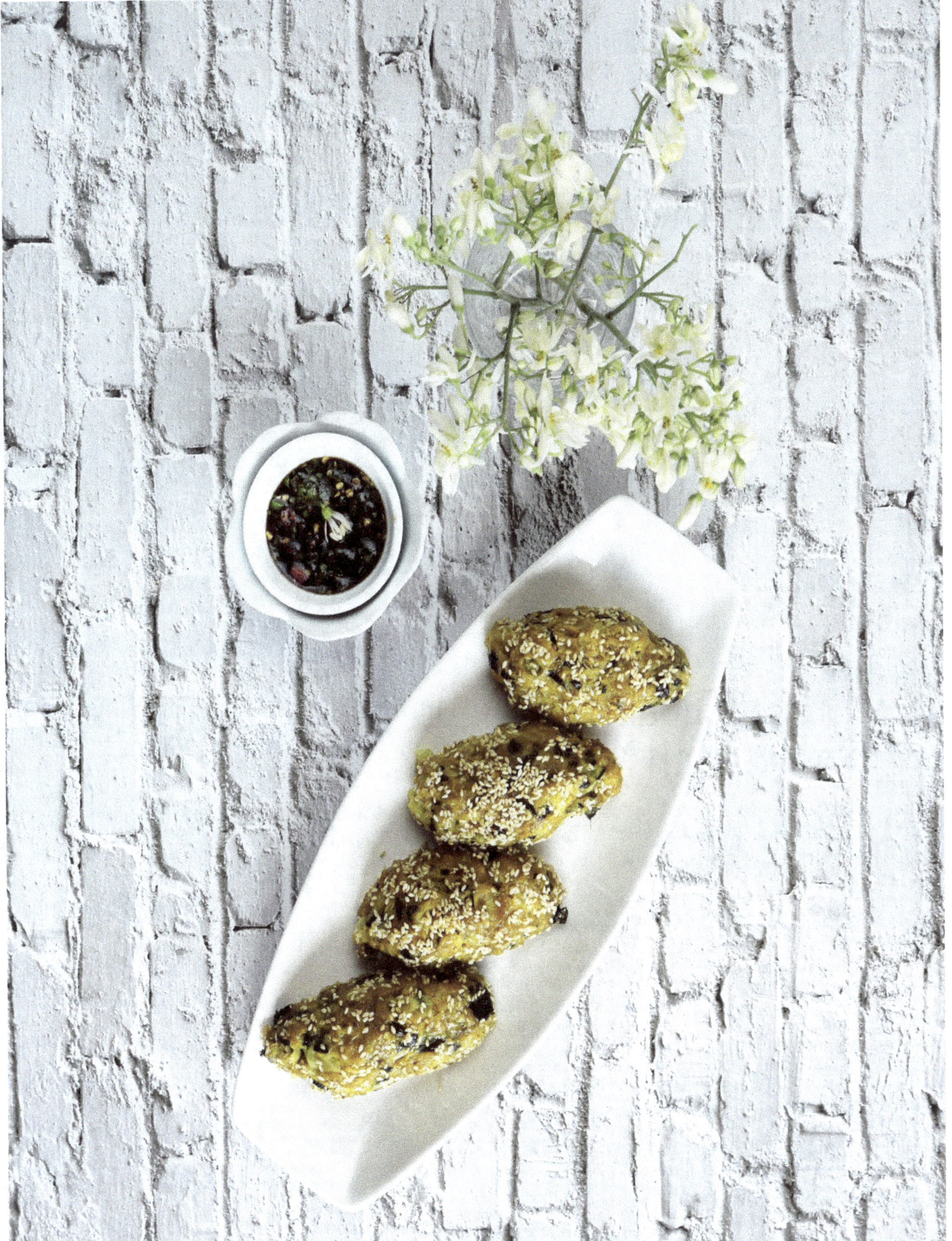

Moringa Tempura

The usual recipe for tempura batter calls for flour, eggs, and ice cold water to give it that light, crispy texture. My secret to keeping it crunchy for hours is to add sparkling water and baking powder.

Ingredients
⅓ cup all-purpose flour
2 tbsp rice flour
2 tbsp corn flour
¼ tsp baking powder
150ml sparkling water, chilled
Salt to taste

Method
1. Wash the moringa leaves and pat dry, leaving the stems intact.
2. Snap the stems with leaves into bite-sized stalks. Set aside.
3. Mix all the dry ingredients in a bowl.
4. Add the chilled sparkling water.
5. Mix well using a whisk.
6. Heat oil in a pan.
7. Dip each bite-sized stalk of moringa leaves in the batter.
8. Drop them carefully in the oil.
9. Deep fry in low heat so as not to change the colour of the batter.
10. Flip and cook briefly.
11. Drain over paper towels
12. Serve hot with Greek Cucumber Yogurt Sauce (recipe below).

Greek Cucumber Yogurt Sauce With Moringa

A popular dip that features in South-Eastern European and Middle Eastern cuisines, it is also known as tzatziki, *cacik*, or *tarator*. The addition of moringa leaves amps up the health benefits of this versatile dip.

Ingredients
1 ½ cups Greek yogurt
1 large cucumber
1 clove garlic
1 tbsp lemon juice
2 tbsp olive oil
2 tbsp fresh dill
1 tbsp fresh mint
1-2 tbsp moringa leaves
Salt to taste
Extra virgin olive oil (to finish)

Method
1. Grate cucumbers.
2. Toss with ½ tsp salt to extract the water.
3. Let sit for 10-15 minutes.
4. Squeeze water from cucumber.
5. Combine all ingredients in a bowl.
6. Taste and season with extra salt, garlic, or lemon juice to suit your taste.
7. Chill before serving.
8. To serve, drizzle with extra virgin olive oil across the top.

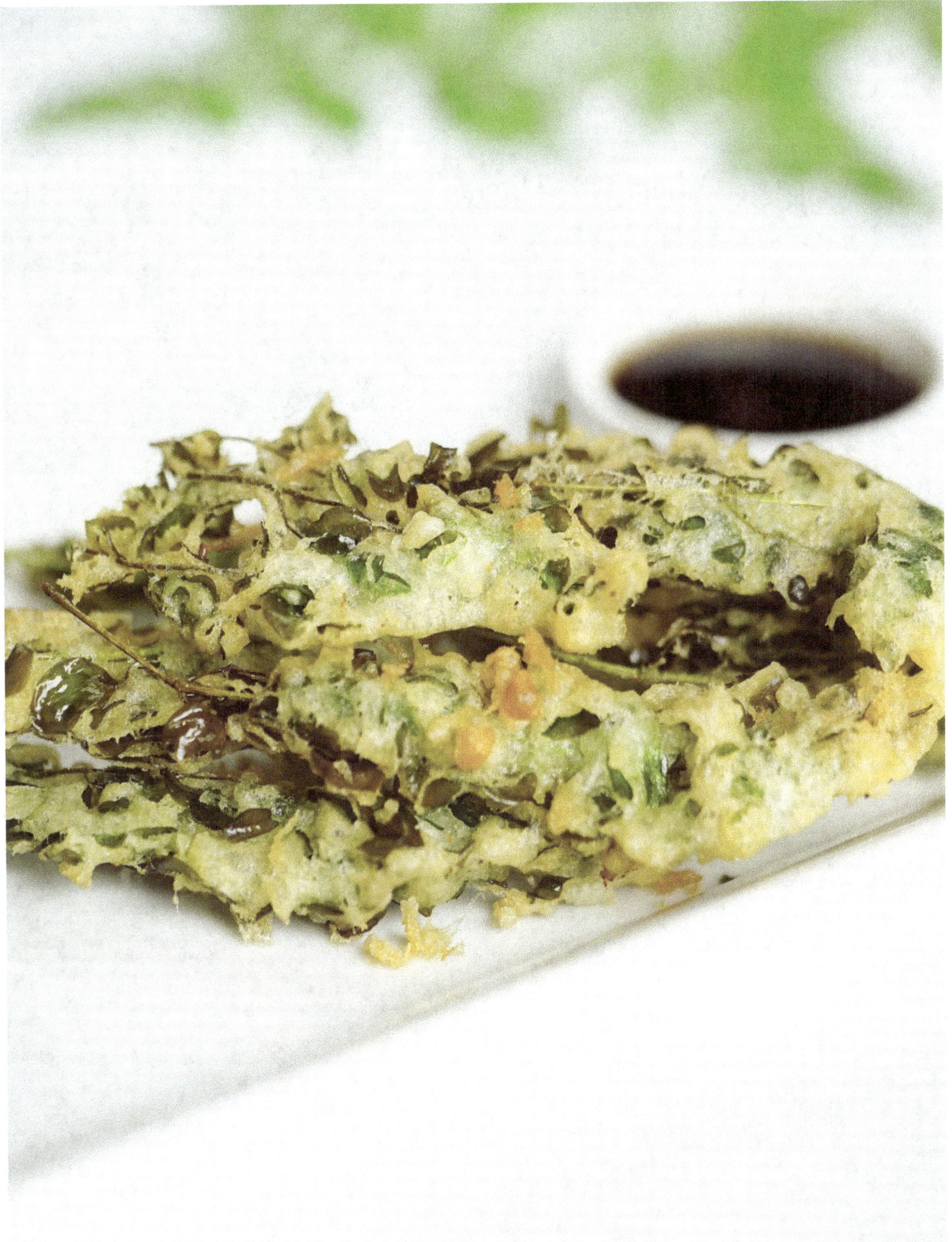

Veggie Moringa Pizza

There are two ways of using moringa leaves when preparing a pizza: add them to the dough, or garnish over the top just before serving. Either way, your pizza will get a superfood boost!

Ingredients (base)
2 ¼ tsp active dry yeast
½ tsp brown sugar
1 ½ cups of warm water
1 tsp salt
2 tbsp oil
3 ⅓ cups all-purpose flour
½ cup moringa leaves, chopped

Method
1. Dissolve yeast and sugar in warm water for 10 minutes.
2. Stir in oil and water.
3. Mix in 3⅓ cups flour and add moringa leaves.
4. Roll and knead the dough until it is no longer sticky.
5. Cover with a warm cloth and keep in a warm area.
6. Let it rise until double the size (about 30-40 minutes).
7. Dough should be smooth and soft.
8. Punch and poke the dough, and let it rise for another 15 minutes.
9. Roll out the dough to the required size.

Ingredients (topping)
2-3 cups shredded mozzarella cheese
1 cup shredded cheese of your choice
1 cup bell peppers, sliced
1 cup mushrooms, sliced
1 cup cherry tomatoes, diced
1 onion, diced
Tomato sauce for base of pizza

Method
1. Pre-heat oven to 425°F/220°C.
2. Spread a thin layer of sauce on the pizza base.
3. Add a layer of your favourite cheese.
4. Place the toppings on top and sprinkle mozzarella cheese over.
5. If you are not using moringa leave in the base, then this is the time to add moringa leaves to the pizza.
6. Bake for 15-20 minutes and serve.

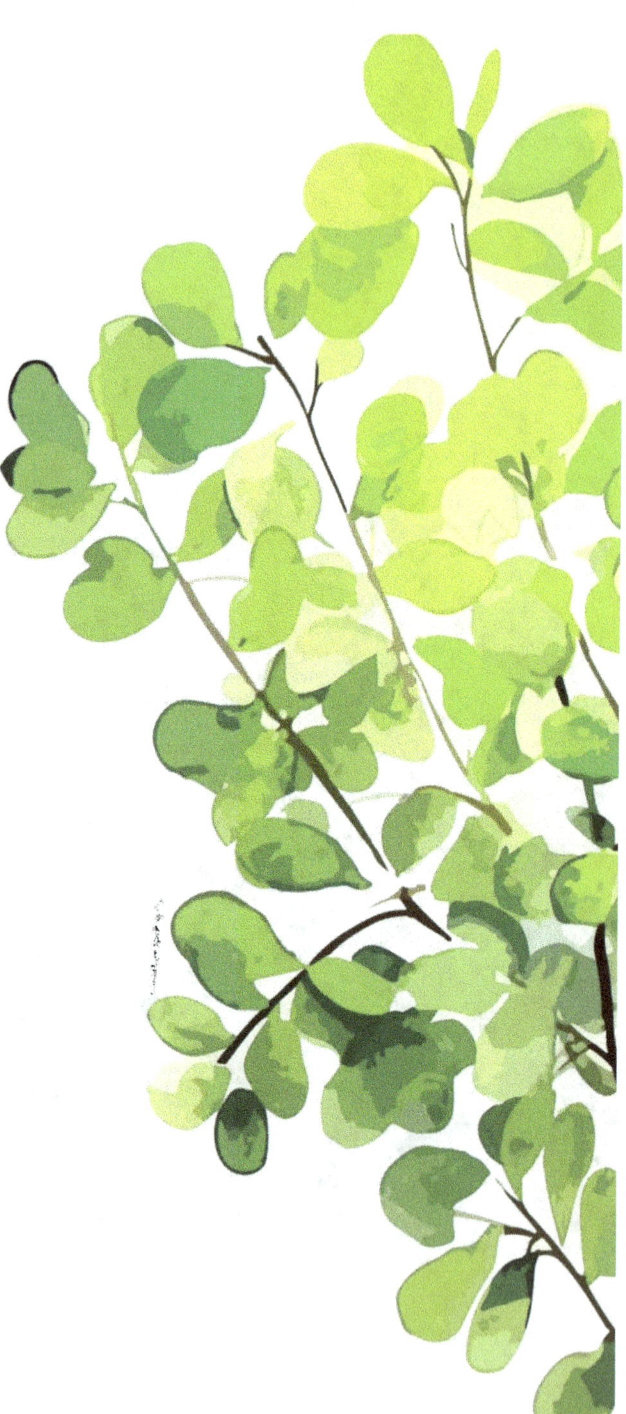

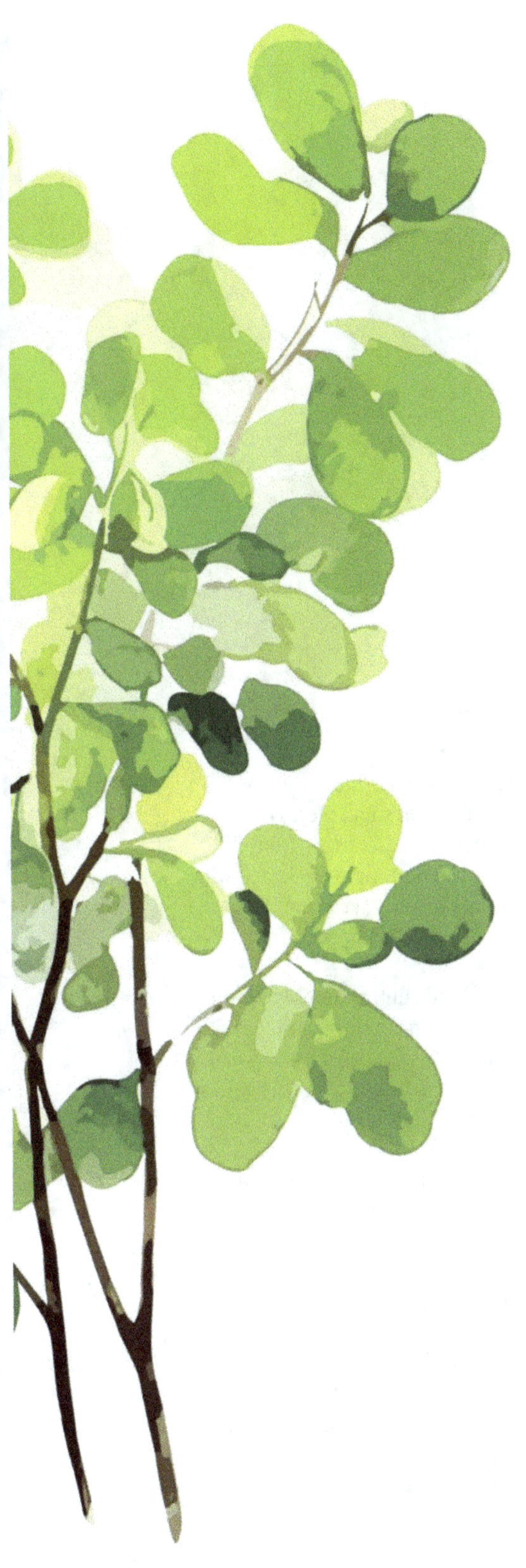

Avocado And Couscous Salad With Moringa Leaves

When you combine moringa leaves with omega 3-rich avocado, you get a wholesome and hearty salad that enriches your body with multiple essential nutrients. Good as a meal on its own or as a side dish.

Ingredients (salad)
2 avocados peeled, stoned and cut into cubes
½ cup couscous
¼ red onion, diced
150gm mozzarella cheese
250gm cherry tomatoes, halved
Handful of moringa leaves
½ cup water
Pine nuts (for garnishing)

Ingredients (dressing)
1 tbsp lemon juice
3 tbsp olive oil
Salt and pepper to taste

Method
1. In a bowl, mix couscous and boiling water.
2. Cover with a plate and leave for five minutes.
3. Mix the dressing.
4. Pour over the couscous and fluff with a fork to ensure it is mixed through.
5. Add the tomatoes, avocado, and mozzarella into the couscous.
6. Stir in the moringa leaves.
7. Garnish with pine nuts and serve.

Moringa Leaf Chaat

Chaat is a family of savoury snacks that originated in India and is usually a delightful combination of salty, spicy, sweet, and sour flavours. This version includes moringa leaves to give it a tinge of herby, nutty taste.

Ingredients
1 cup moringa leaves
½ cup raw peanuts
2 tsp tamarind chutney*
2 tbsp oil
Salt to taste
1 tsp green chutney*
3 medium potatoes
1 tsp *chaat masala* powder*
1 tsp lemon juice
1 medium carrot, grated
1 medium chilli

For garnishing
1 cup coriander leaves, chopped
½ cup *sev**

Method
1. Heat some oil in a shallow pan.
2. Add the moringa leaves and fry on high flame until they lose their moisture and turn crispy.
3. Transfer them onto a plate lined with absorbent paper.
4. Dry roast the peanuts and set aside.
5. Boil the potatoes and peel them. Set aside.
6. Grate the carrots and set aside.
7. Mix potatoes, peanuts, *chaat* masala powder, tamarind chutney, lemon juice, coriander leaves, *sev*, carrots, salt, and the fried moringa leaves.
8. Add chopped green chillies.
9. Place the *chaat* in a serving bowl.
10. Top with the green chutney and some tamarind chutney.
11. Sprinkle some *sev* over.
12. Serve garnished with pomegranate seeds and drizzled with curd.

***Notes:**
Sev is a popular Indian snack consisting of small pieces of crunchy noodles made from chickpea flour paste seasoned with turmeric, salt, cayenne and carom seeds before being deep-fried.

Tamarind chutney is a sweet and sour Indian condiment made with tamarind, salt, jaggery, and ground spices. It is readily available at East Asian food stores.

Green chutney is a delicious mix of fresh coriander, mint leaves, cumin, ginger, garlic, lemon juice, green chillies, and salt. It is readily available at East Asian food stores.

Chaat masala is a lovely spice blend that adds hints of saltiness, spiciness, and zestiness to any dish you add it to. It is readily available at East Asian food stores.

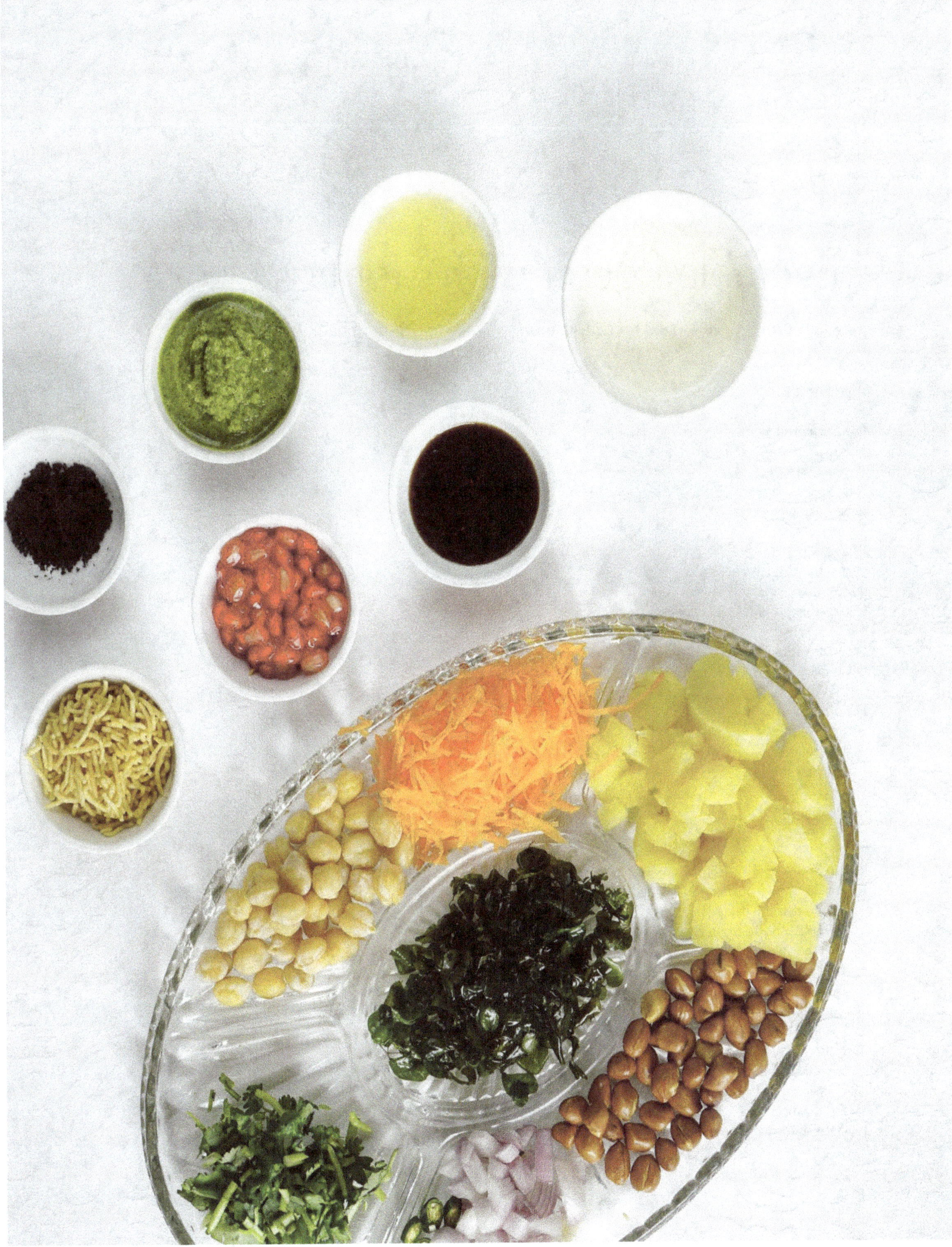

Vegetable Pajeon With Moringa

We transform the well-loved Korean scallion pancake into a moringa-infused delight!

Ingredients

For the pancake
½ cup all-purpose flour
½ potato starch
Salt to taste
½ tsp baking powder
¾ cup ice water
1 large egg
¼ cup onion, finely chopped
4 cups mixed vegetable of your choice
(e.g. carrots, zucchini, bell peppers,) finely chopped
4 scallions, thinly sliced
½ cup moringa leaves
Oil as needed

For dipping sauce
3 tbsp soy sauce
2 tsp rice vinegar
1 tsp grated ginger
½ tsp sesame oil
Pinch of sugar
Salt to taste

Method
1. For the pancake balter, whisk together all-purpose flour, potato starch, salt, and baking powder.
2. In another bowl, combine water, egg, and onions.
3. Add the mixture to the pancake batter and whisk until smooth.
4. Fold in vegetables and ¾ of the scallions.
5. Heat a large non-stick skillet over medium heat.
6. Add a little oil.
7. Scoop ¼ cup portions of batter onto the skillet.
8. Flatten and fry for 2-3 minutes.
9. Flip and add moringa leaves, then continue to fry until browned.
10. Transfer to a plate lined with paper towels.
11. For the dip, mix together all the ingredients.
12. Garnish the pancakes with sliced scallions and serve with the dip.

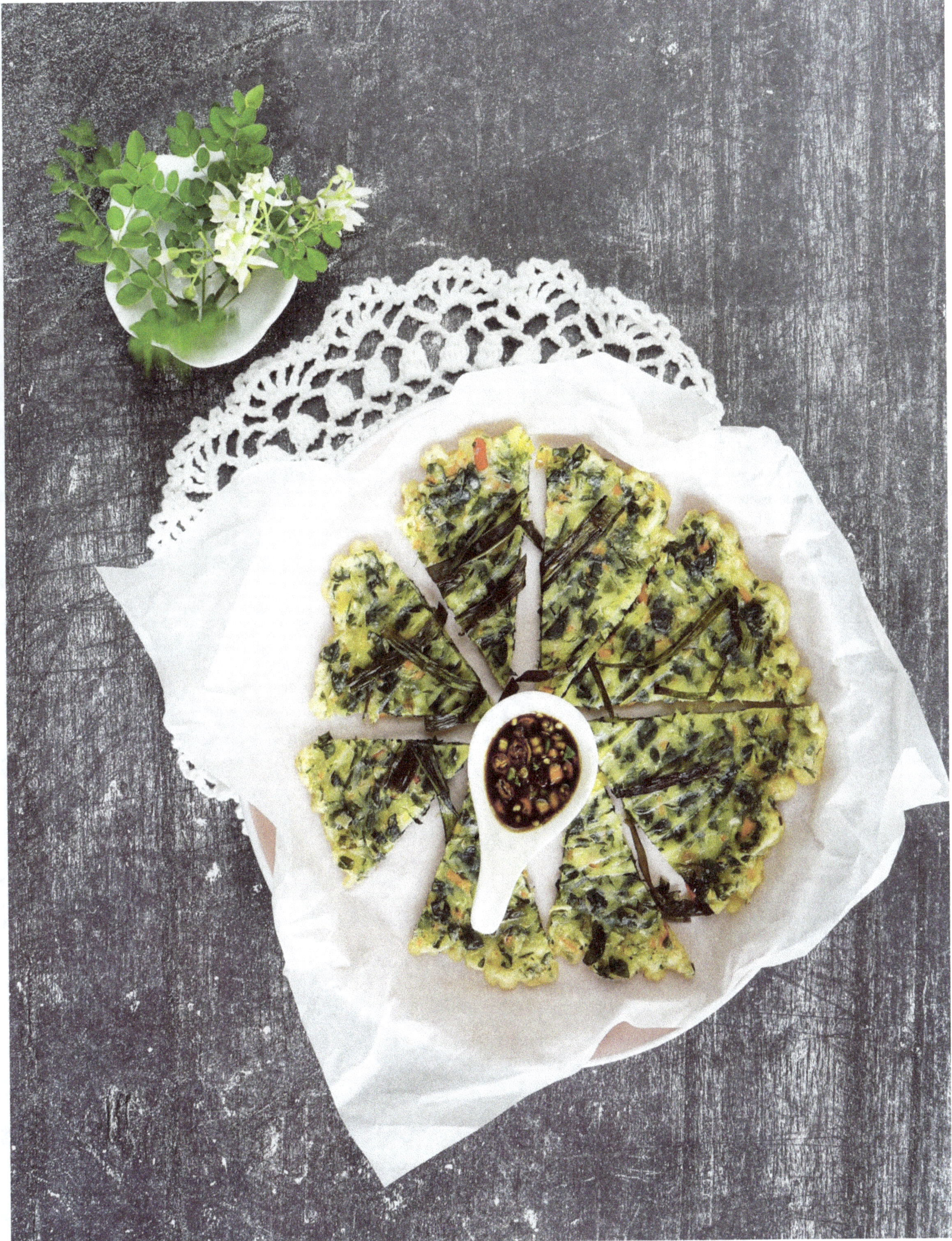

Moringa Minestrone Soup

Level up the classic Italian-style minestrone by adding moringa leaves.

Ingredients

For the barley
½ cup pearled barley
2 cups water
1 tsp oil

For the vegetable broth
1 cup celery, diced
1 cup onion, diced
1 cup carrots, diced
Salt to taste
2 cloves garlic, chopped
1 litre water

For the minestrone
6 cups vegetable broth
2 cups ripe tomatoes, diced
½ cup fresh corn kernels
1 ½ cups cooked kidney beans
1 cup cabbage, coarsley chopped
2 large sage leaves
4 sprigs fresh thyme
3 small bay leaves

For garnishing
2 cups fresh moringa leaves

Method
(Barley)
1. Boil two cups of water.
2. Add the barley.
3. Reduce heat and cook until tender.

(Vegetable broth)
1. Heat oil in a soup pot.
2. Add the celery, onions, and carrots. Sauté until the onions turn soft and brown.
3. Add salt and garlic.
4. Add water and bring to a boil. Turn down heat, cover, and let simmer for about 60 minutes.

(Minestrone)
1. In a soup pot, add vegetable broth, tomatoes, corn, beans, cabbage, sage, thyme, bay leaves, and the cooked barley with its cooking water.
2. Boil over low heat for 15 minutes.
3. Add moringa leaves and cook for a few minutes.
4. Remove bay leaves, sage leaves, and thyme sprigs from the soup.
5. Serve hot with Pandesal Buns (see recipe on pg 72).

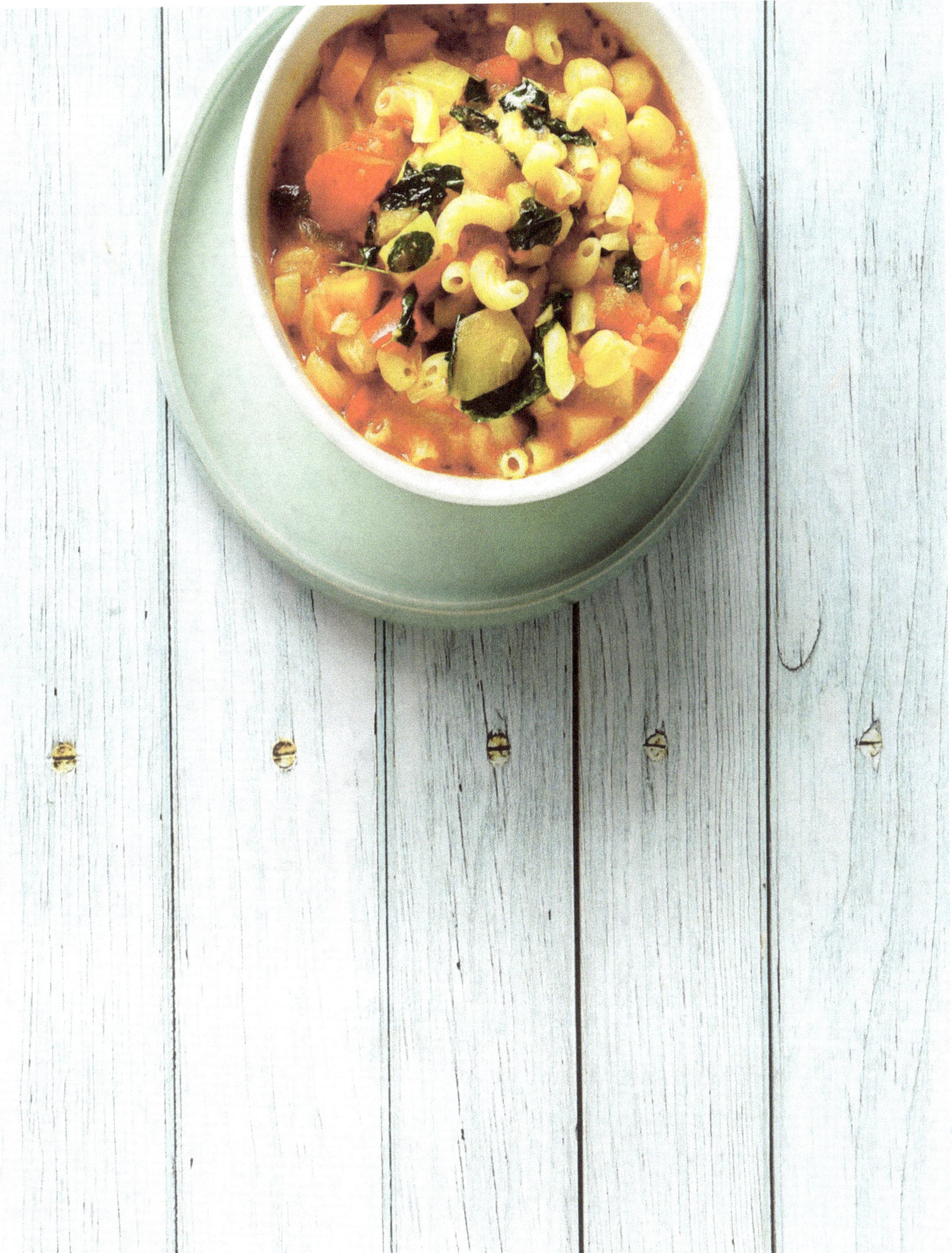

Moringa Leaves In Coconut Milk

Hearty, wholesome and so easy to make, this recipe is set to become a favourite among the whole family.

Ingredients
3 cups moringa leaves
1 onion, thinly sliced
1 clove garlic, crushed
200ml coconut milk

Method
1. Put the coconut milk, onion and garlic in a pot.
2. Simmer over low heat.
3. Once the onion caramelizes, add moringa leaves and the seasoning.
4. Simmer again for about 10 minutes on low heat.
5. Serve hot. Best enjoyed with rice.

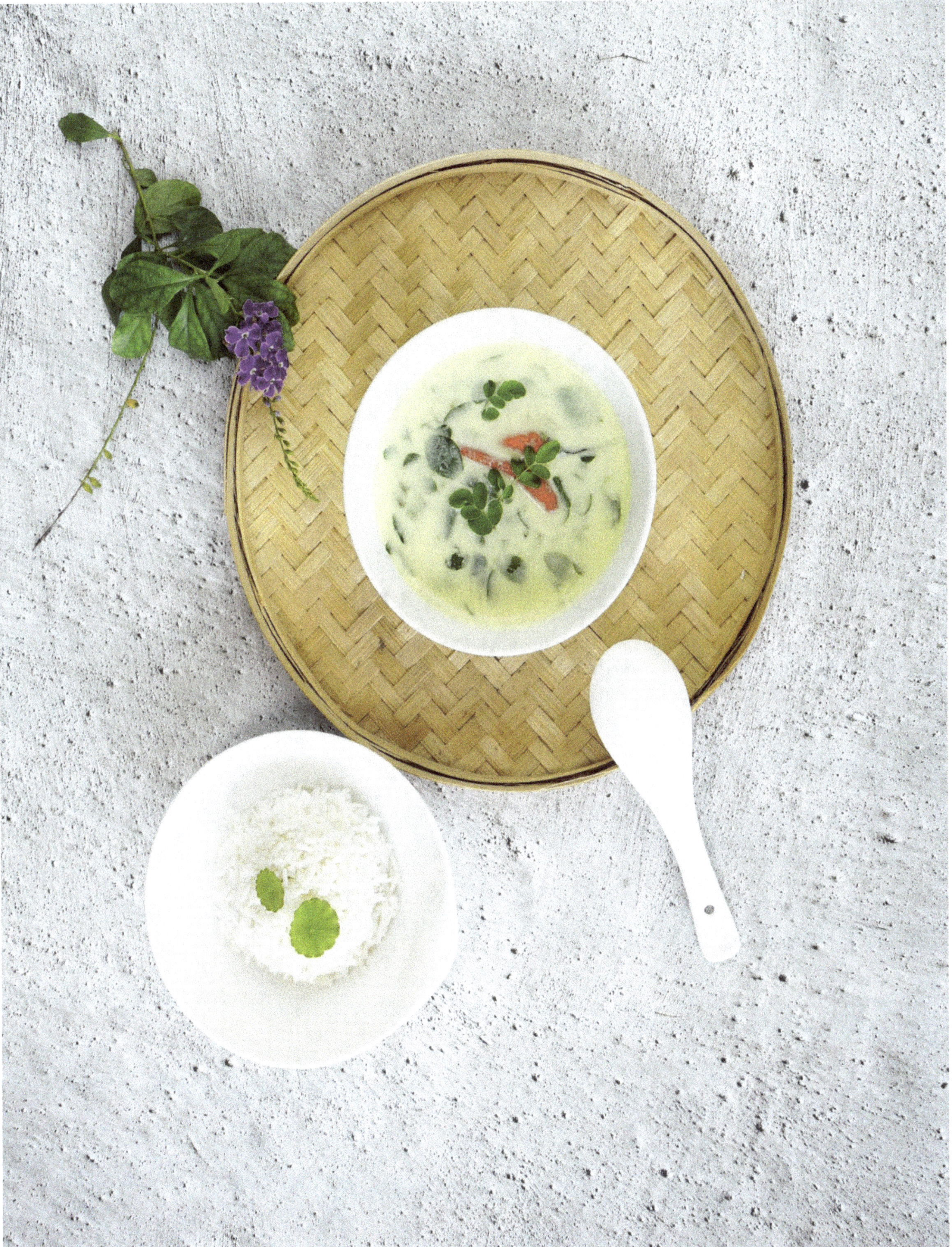

Miso Moringa Noodle Soup

Moringa leaves blend beautifully with rich miso into a light, gingery broth that's power-packed with umami notes. This nourishing noodle soup is soothing and comforting.

Ingredients

300gm noodles of your choice
5 cups vegetable broth, or stock water or combination
1 inch piece of ginger, grated
1 medium zucchini, shredded
1 bell pepper, thinly sliced
4 tbsp miso (any variety)
1 tsp chilli garlic sauce
½ cup moringa leaves
2-3 spring onions (white and light green parts only), finely chopped

Method

1. Cook noodles according to instructions on packaging.
2. Place broth, ginger, and vegetables in a stockpot.
3. Bring to a near boil and simmer for approximately 5 minutes.
4. On medium low heat, stir in miso paste, chilli garlic sauce, and moringa leaves
5. Simmer gently for a further 2 minutes.
6. Divide cooked noodles into bowls and ladle soup on top.
7. Garnish with sliced spring onions and serve.

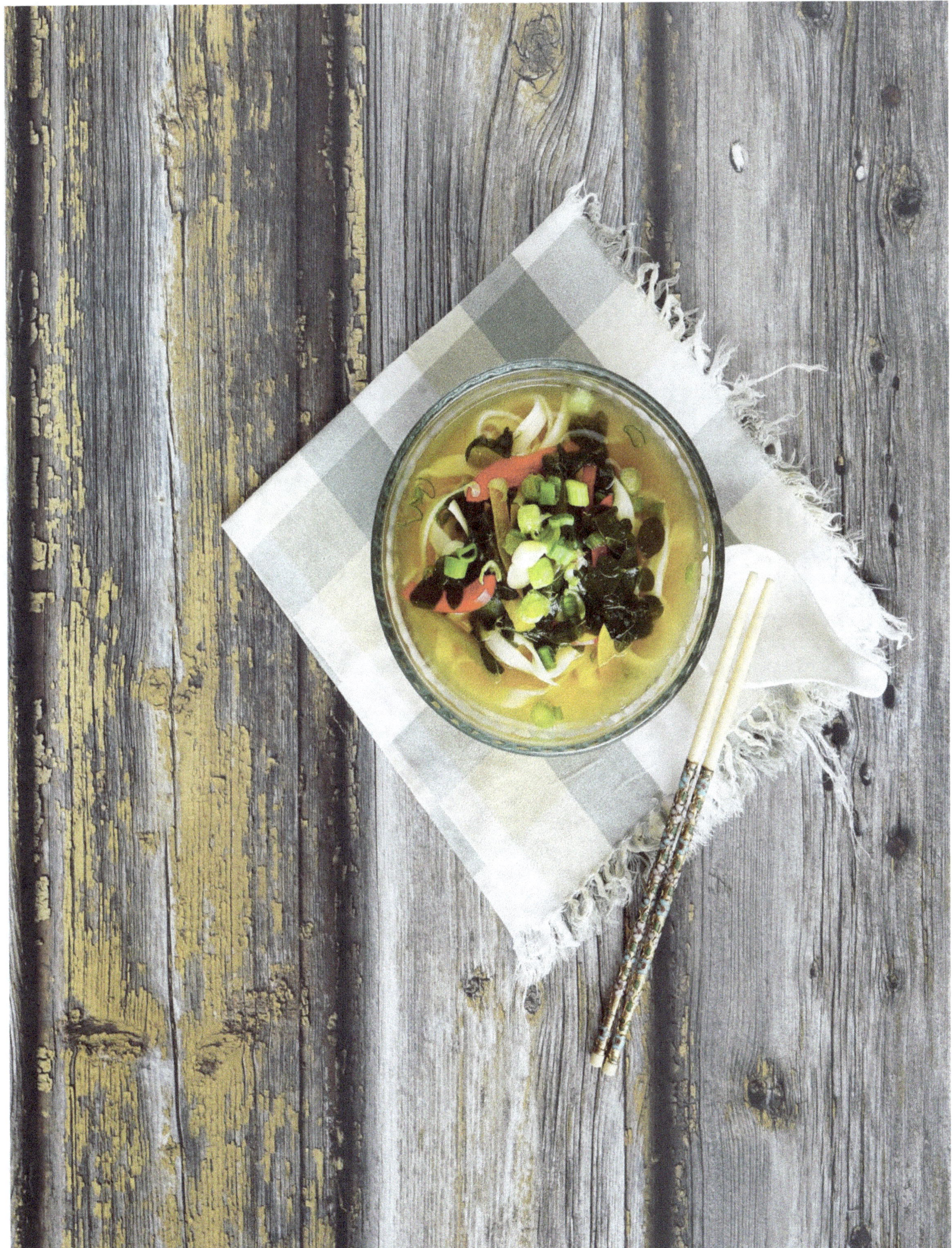

Filipino Corn And Moringa Soup

Enjoy the sweetness of the corn and the savoury, slightly nutty goodness of fresh moringa leaves in a bowl. My Filipino helpers, Lyn and Christine, were the ones who introduced me to this simple, comforting soup.

Ingredients
1 ½ cups corn kernels
1 cup moringa leaves
2-3 cups chicken or vegetable broth
2 tsp minced garlic
1 small onion, chopped
2 tbsp oil
Salt and pepper to taste

Method
1. Heat a cooking pot and pour in the oil.
2. When hot, sauté the garlic and onion.
3. Add the corn and stir.
4. Pour in the broth and bring to a boil.
5. Simmer for 8-10 minutes.
6. Add the moringa leaves.
7. Stir and simmer for two minutes.
8. Turn off heat.
9. Transfer to a serving bowl.
10. Serve hot.

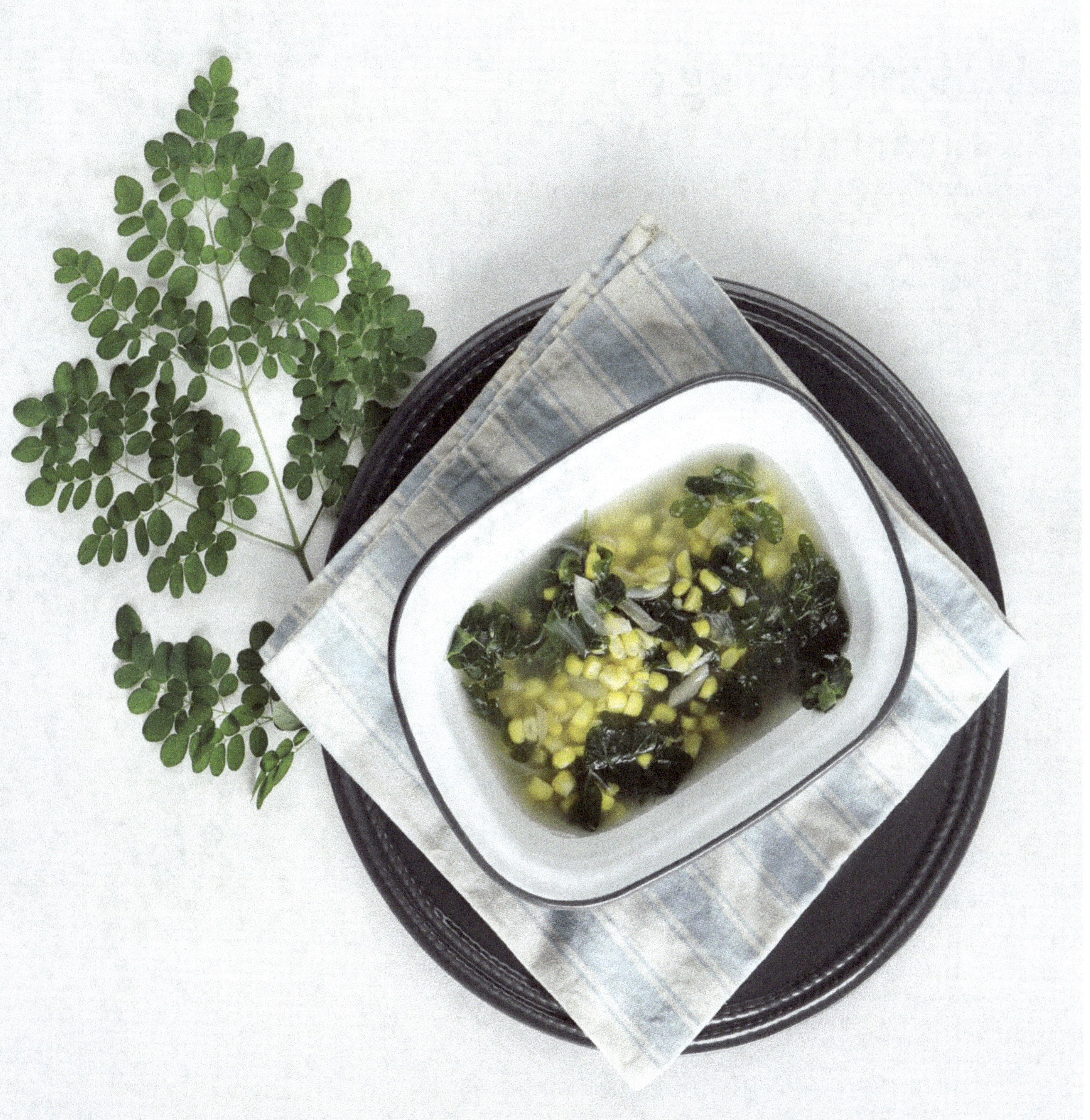

Moringa Veggie Enchilada

Add a touch of moringa to this classic Mexican delight.

Ingredients

8-10 small soft corn tortillas
2 cups moringa leaves, chopped
1 can (16oz/450gm) of black beans
1 can (16oz/450gm) of tomatoes
1 can (16oz/450gm) of corn
1 can (14oz/400gm) of green salsa
1 hot pepper
½ tsp cumin
½ tsp chilli powder
½ tsp paprika
½ tsp grated garlic
1 medium onion, chopped
2 medium bell peppers, chopped
2 tbsp oil
2 cups shredded cheese (Mexican blend or Monterey jack)
¼ chopped cilantro
¼ cup chopped spring onion

Method

1. Pre-heat oven to 375°F/190°C.
2. In a large skillet, sauté onions in 1 tbsp oil.
3. Add bell peppers and sauté for a few minutes.
4. Add corn, beans, tomatoes, and green salsa.
5. Stir in the spices.
6. Bring the mixture to a simmer for about 10 minutes.
7. Remove from pan and stir in chopped moringa leaves.

To assemble

1. Oil a large casserole dish.
2. Place a layer of tortillas.
3. Layer veggie mixture over.
4. Sprinkle with cheese.
5. Add next layer of tortillas, veggie mixture, and cheese.
6. Continue to layer until you are out of veggie mixture.
7. Finish with cheese on top.
8. Bake for 15-20 minutes or until cheese starts to bubble and brown.
9. Allow to cool.
10. Garnish with chopped cilantro and spring onion, and serve.

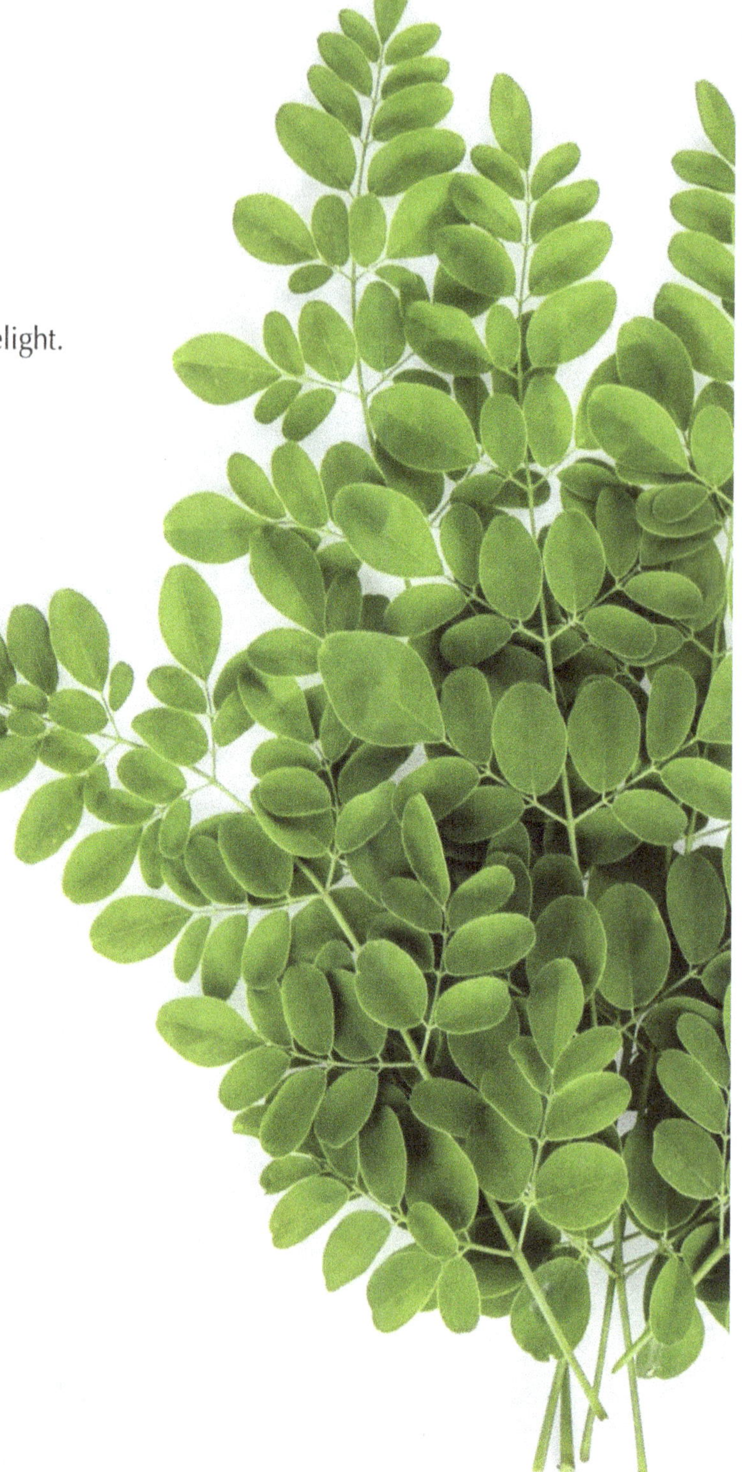

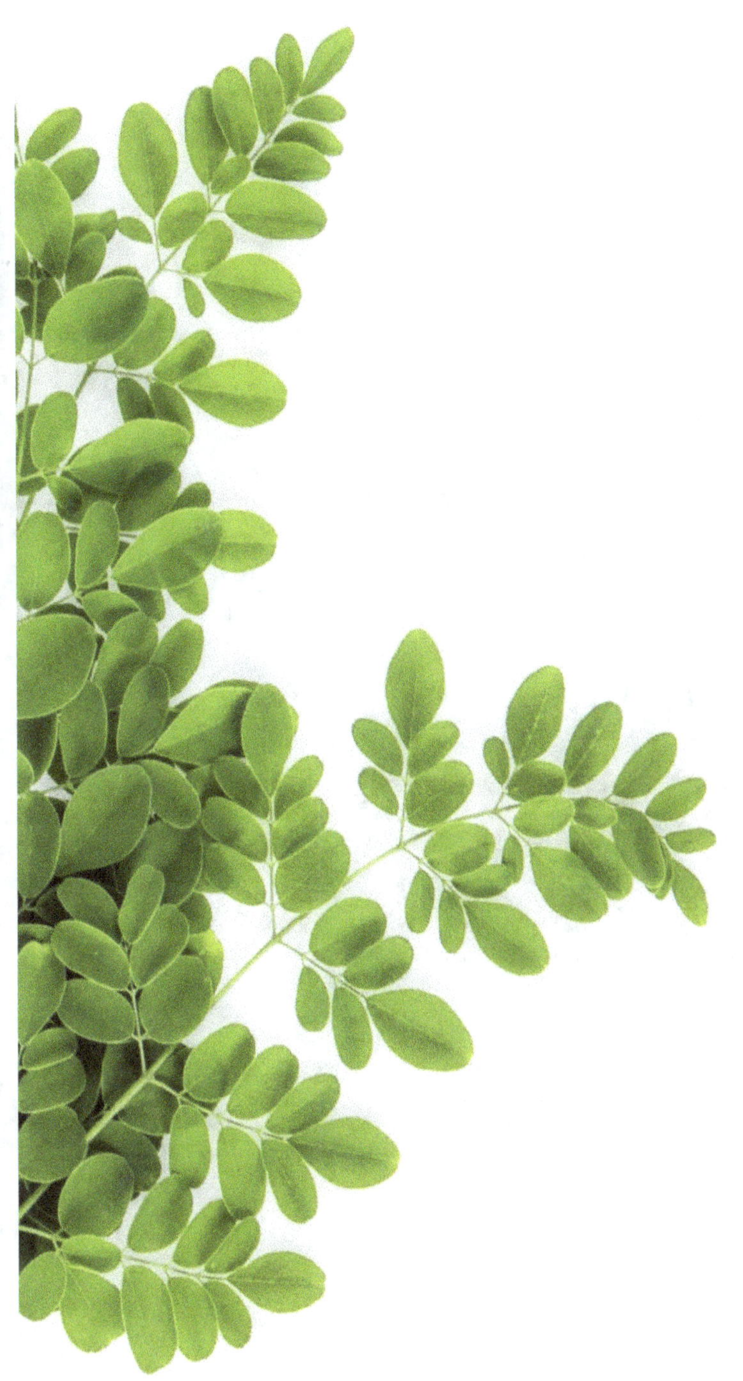

Egg Rolls With Moringa Leaves

Soft, fluffy, cheesy omelette packed with the goodness of moringa leaves are ideal for a healthy, hearty breakfast.

Ingredients

4 eggs
1 tbsp all-purpose four
Salt and pepper to taste
2 green chillies, finely chopped
¼ cup cheddar cheese
1 cup moringa leaves, finely chopped
Butter or oil for cooking

Method

1. Pre-heat the oven to 180°C/356°F.
2. Line a baking pan and grease it with butter.
3. Heat a teaspoon of oil in a small pan.
4. Add the moringa leaves, sprinkle salt, and cook until the leaves wilt and all the excess moisture evaporates.
5. Allow the moringa leaves to cool.
6. Whisk the eggs along with the flour, salt, pepper and green chillies.
7. Pour egg mixture into the prepared pan.
8. Sprinkle cheddar cheese on top.
9. Cover the pan and bake the egg mixture until it sets.
10. Once the egg has set, remove from the oven and allow to cool.
11. Loosen the egg mixture from the sides of the pan and carefully roll up, jelly-roll fashion.
12. Garnish with fresh moringa leaves to serve.

Moringa Smoothie With Milk, Pineapple, Banana And Chia Seeds

Smoothies are a quick and easy way to consume a large amount of vegetables, fruits, and herbs at one go. And the best part is, you can mix and match the ingredients to your liking. Remember to add a handful of fresh moringa leaves into your blend!

Ingredients
1 cup milk of your choice (dairy or non-dairy)
½ cup fresh moringa leaves/2 tsp moringa powder
1 banana, cut into chunks
½ cup pineapple
1 tbsp chia seeds

Method
1. Soak chia seeds for 20-30 minutes.
2. In the base of a high-speed blender, combine the milk, moringa leaves, banana, and pineapple.
3. Blend on high for 30-45 seconds or until the smoothie is thick and creamy.
4. Pour into a glass.
5. The chia seeds should turn gelatinous by now. Stir into the smoothie.
6. Serve immediately.

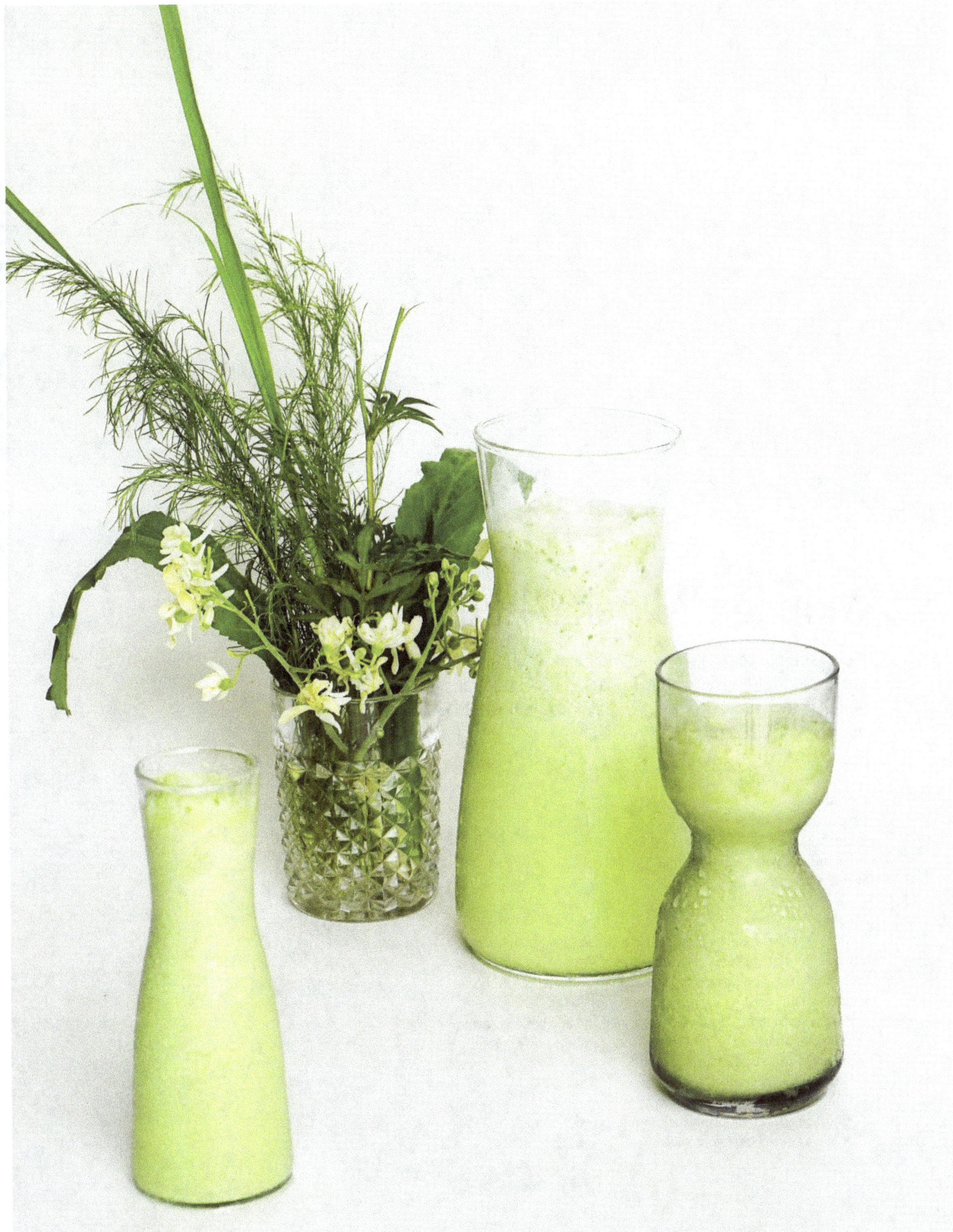

Moringa 'Matcha' Latte

Here's an interesting fact about moringa: when the dried leaves are ground into powder, the aroma and taste are similar to matcha! You can use moringa powder like you would matcha to whip up milky, comforting green lattes.

Ingredients
1 tsp moringa powder
¼ cup hot water
¼ cup milk of your choice, warmed
Sweetener of choice (optional)

Method
1. Moringa powder can be clumpy. Use a *chasen* (bamboo matcha whisk) to sift the clumps into fine powder.
2. If you don't have a *chasen*, you can also use a strainer to sift the moringa powder.
3. Put the sifted moringa powder into a mug and add boiling water. Whisk vigorously in an up-down motion until the powder is fully dissolved and the mixture is foamy.
4. Pour the warmed milk into the mixture.
5. Whisk again to get the milk frothy.
6. Enjoy it as is, with a sprinkle of moringa powder over the top, or add a sweetener of your choice.

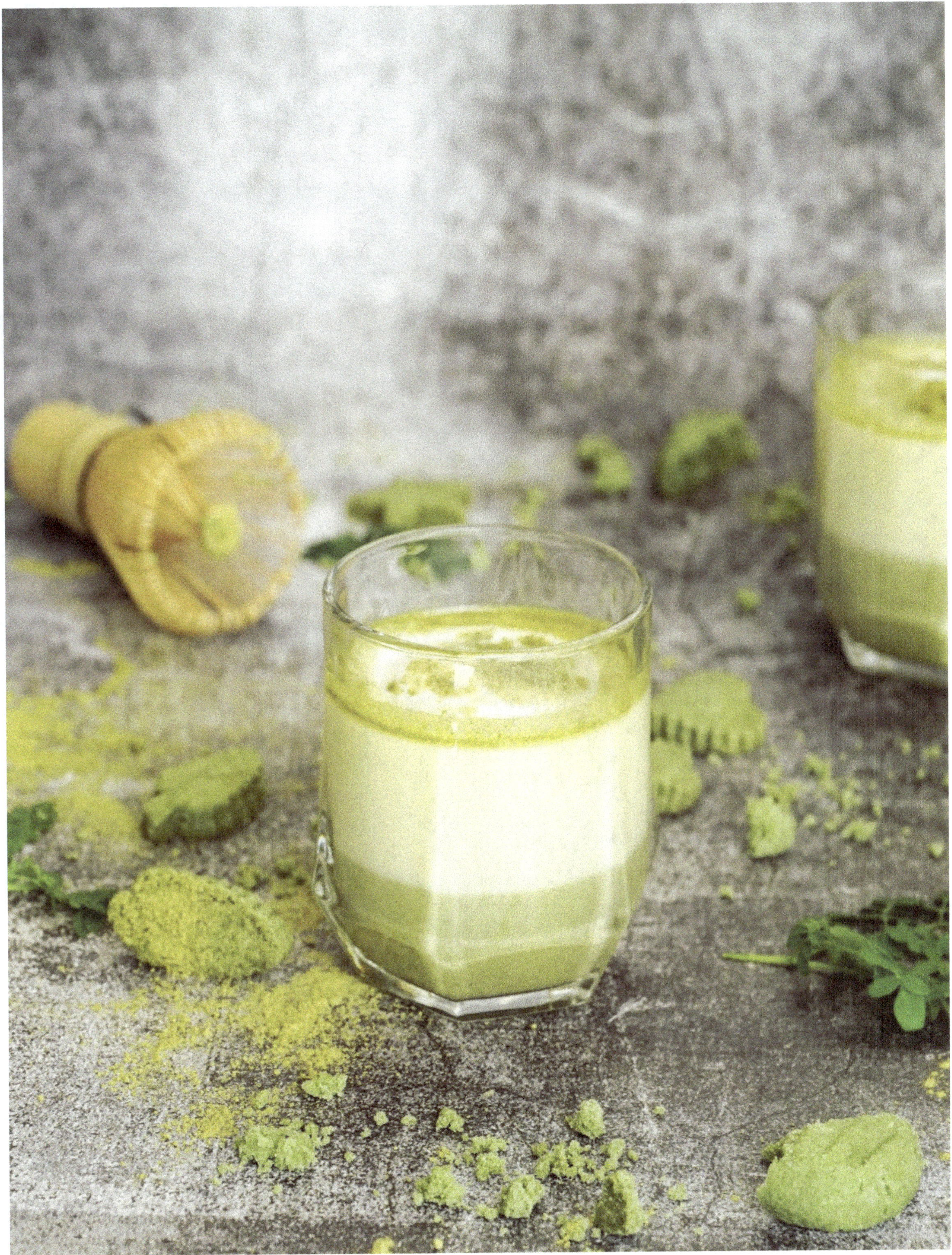

Moringa Iced Teas

All you have to do is steep some moringa leaves in hot water, then chill, and flavour with your choice of fresh herbs and fruits.

Ingredients
Handful of moringa leaves*
2 tsp honey, or any natural sweetener of choice (optional)
Ice cubes
Fresh herbs or fresh fruits, sliced or cut into cubes (to flavour the tea)

Can be replaced with 1 tbsp moringa powder

Method
1. Place the moringa leaves into a teapot and pour boiling water over. Let it steep for 5 minutes.
2. Let cool.
3. To serve, place ice cubes in serving glasses along with your choice of herbs or fruits.
4. If you like your tea sweet, add honey or any natural sweetener.

Tip You can also freeze moringa leaves or flowers into ice cubes and use them to keep the teas cold!

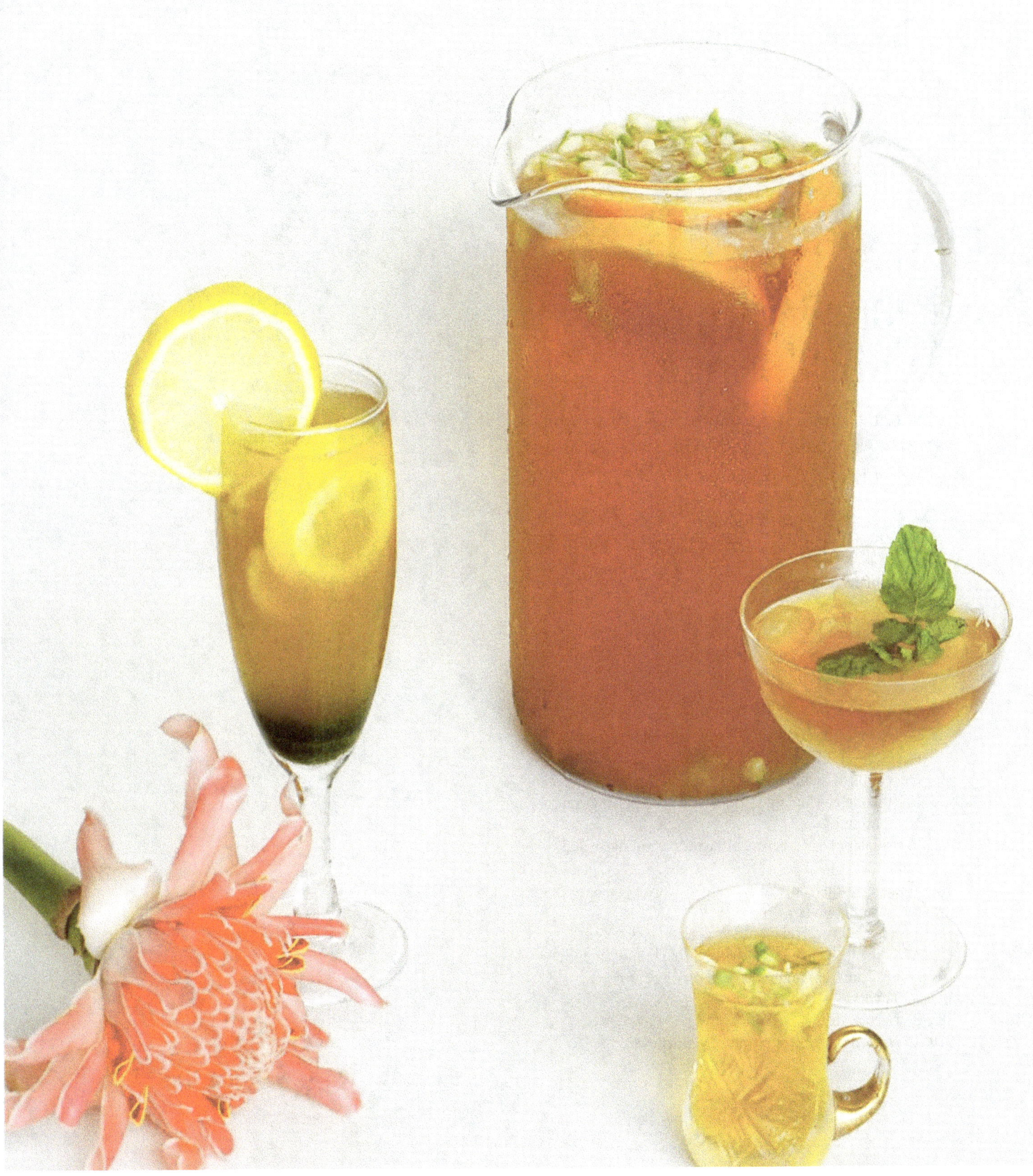

Panna Cotta With Moringa

One of the quickest and easiest desserts to whip up at home, the panna cotta can be made ahead and last for a few days if stored well in the refrigerator.

Ingredients
¼ cup milk
1 ¼ tsp unflavoured gelatin
2 cups heavy cream
¼ cup sugar
1 tsp vanilla essence
1 cup fresh moringa leaves

Method
1. Boil the moringa leaves in a small amount of water for 2-3 minutes.
2. Once cooked, remove the leaves and puree. Set aside.
3. In a mixing bowl, place the milk and gelatin. Let stand for 10-15 minutes.
4. In a small pot or saucepan, place the cream, sugar, and vanilla.
5. Using medium heat, slowly bring mixture a boil or until the sugar dissolves.
6. Stir in gelatin and milk until the gelatin is dissolved.
7. Add the moringa puree and mix through until smooth.
8. Pour the mixture into individual serving cups or containers.
9. Refrigerate for 2-4 hours or until set.
10. To serve, top with fresh fruits of your choice.

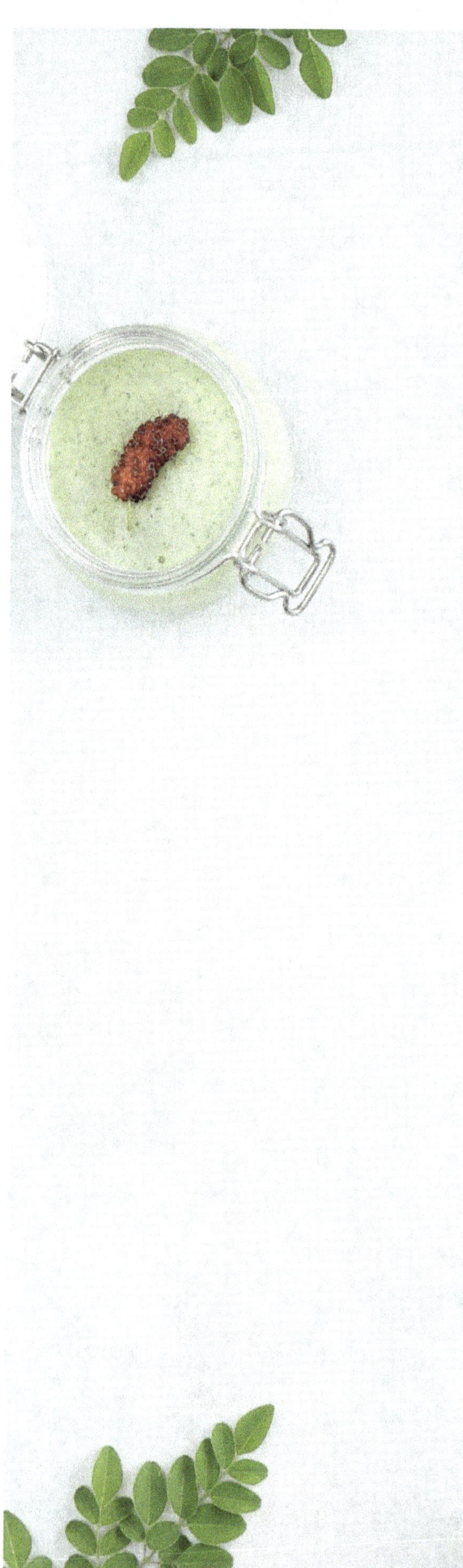

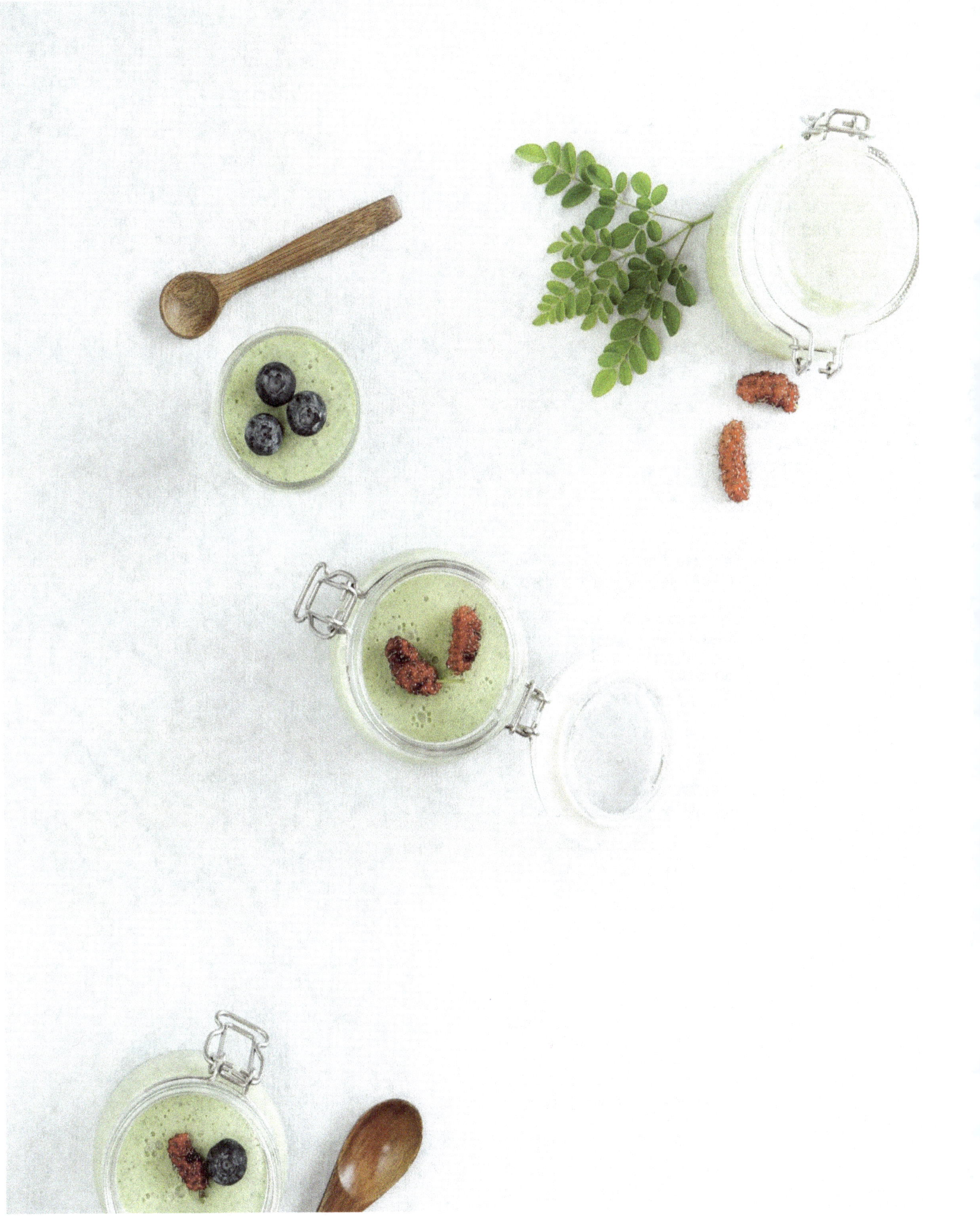

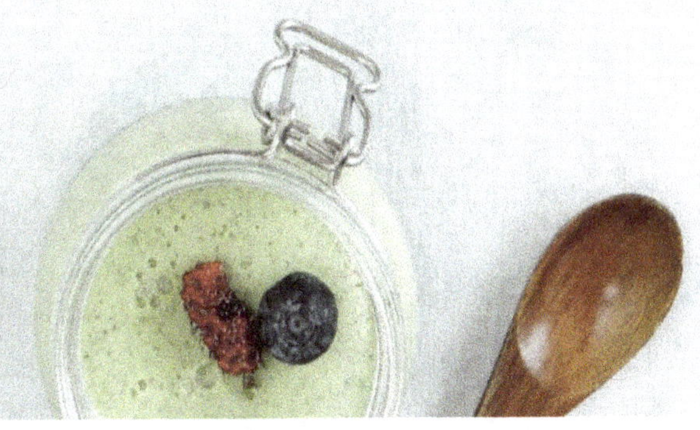

Moringa Macarons

Bite into one of these delicate French delights and savour the sensation of the crispy almond-rich, moringa-infused shells giving way to more moringa goodness in the smooth, creamy filling.

Ingredients (macaron shells)
Whites of 2 eggs (AA size)
¾ cup almond flour
1 cup icing sugar
¼ cup castor sugar
1 tsp moringa powder

Ingredients (filling)
150gm cream cheese
¼ cup icing sugar
⅓ cup whipping cream
1 tbsp moringa powder

Method
1. In a medium mixing bowl, beat the egg whites with an electric hand mixer on medium speed until soft peaks form.
2. Add ½ of the castor sugar and with mixer on high and continue to beat until egg whites are stiff peaks.
3. Repeat with the remaining sugar, beating until whites are shiny and fluffy.
4. With a fine mesh strainer, sieve the almond flour, powdered sugar, and moringa powder into the bowl with the egg whites. Discard any large pieces that remain in the strainer.
5. Fold until just combined.
6. Fill a piping bag with the macaron mixture and pipe 1 ½-inch (4cm) dollops onto a parchment paper-lined baking sheet.
7. Let the cookies rest until they are no longer wet to the touch and a skin forms on top (this can take up to 1 hour).
8. When the cookies are dry to the touch or a skin has formed on the shells, bake at 248°F/120°C for 20 minutes.
9. While the cookies are resting, make the filling by mixing cream cheese, powdered sugar, whipping cream, and moringa powder until smooth.
10. Transfer to a piping bag and set aside until ready to fill.
11. Let rest for 10 minutes, or until mixture has cooled before filling.
12. Pipe the cream cheese mixture onto the flat side of the macaron shell and sandwich with another one.

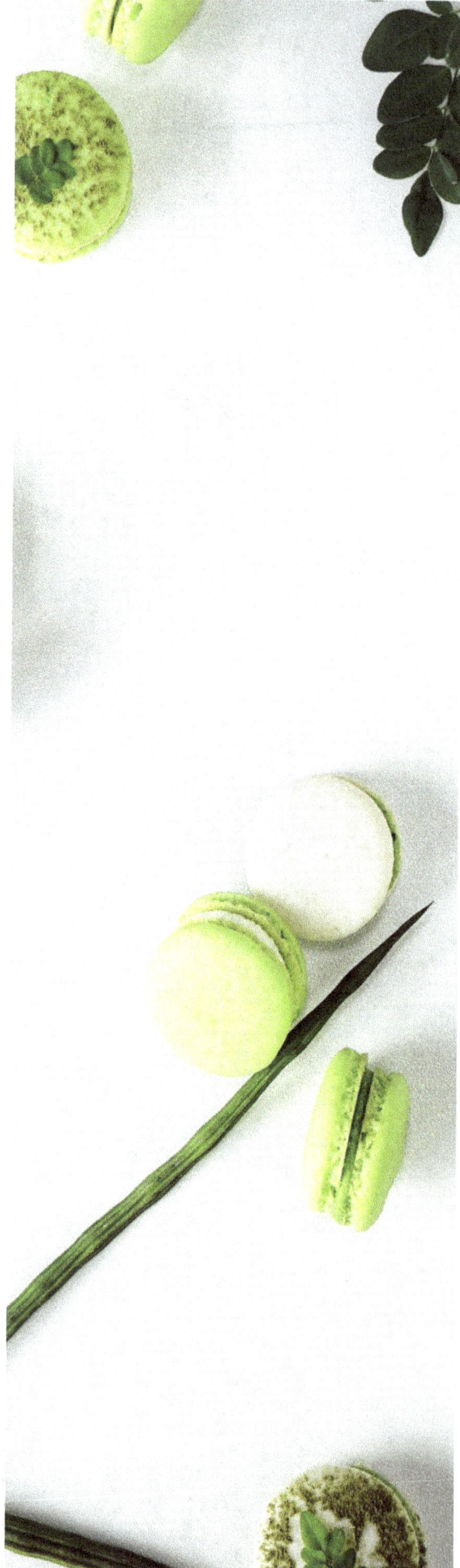

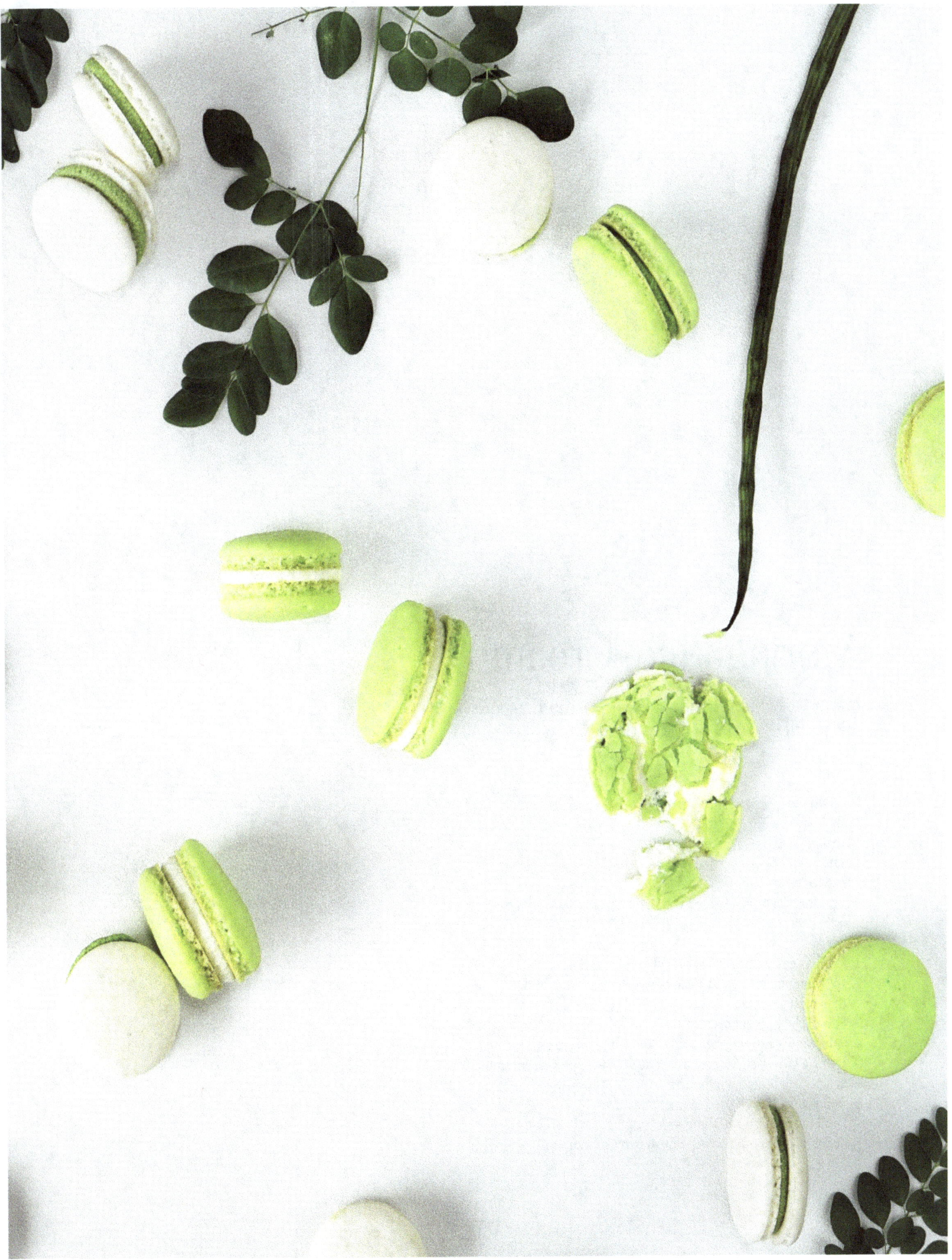

Moringa Ice-Cream

Immortalise the superfood powers of moringa into this joyful dessert that the whole family will enjoy!

Ingredients
1 cup heavy cream
1 tsp vanilla extract
1 can sweetened condensed milk
2 tbsp topping of your choice
1 cup moringa leaves, blitzed with a bit of water to form a paste

Method
1. Whip the heavy cream until stiff peaks appear.
2. In a separate bowl, add 1 can of sweetened condensed milk and the moringa paste.
3. Stir all the ingredients.
4. Add vanilla extract, then fold in the whipped cream.
5. Using a whisk, stir the mixture with the whipped cream until everything is mixed together.
6. Transfer mixture to a container and cover.
7. Chill in freezer for 8-12 hours.
8. Serve in cones or cups. Add fresh fruits as toppings if you wish.

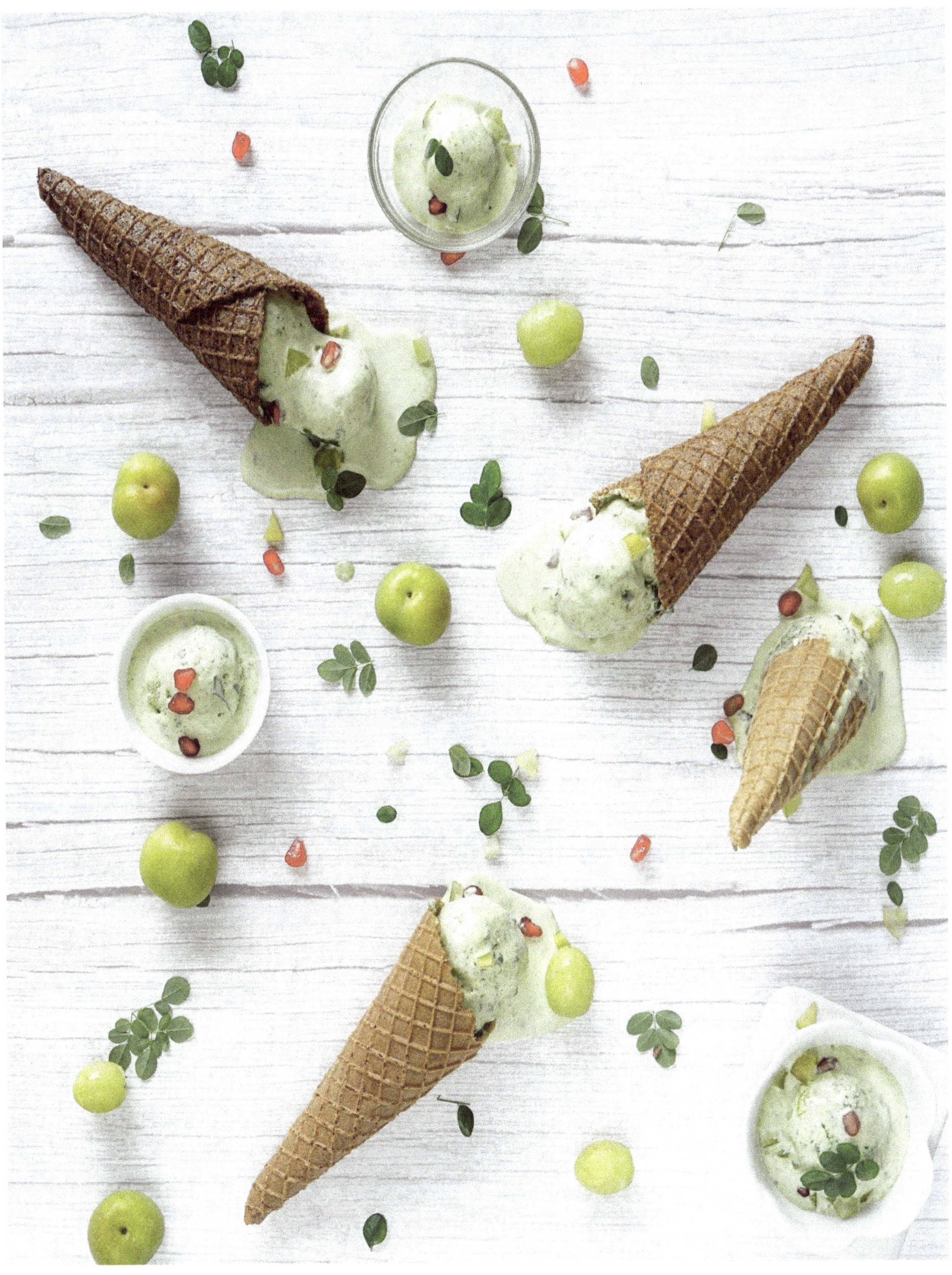

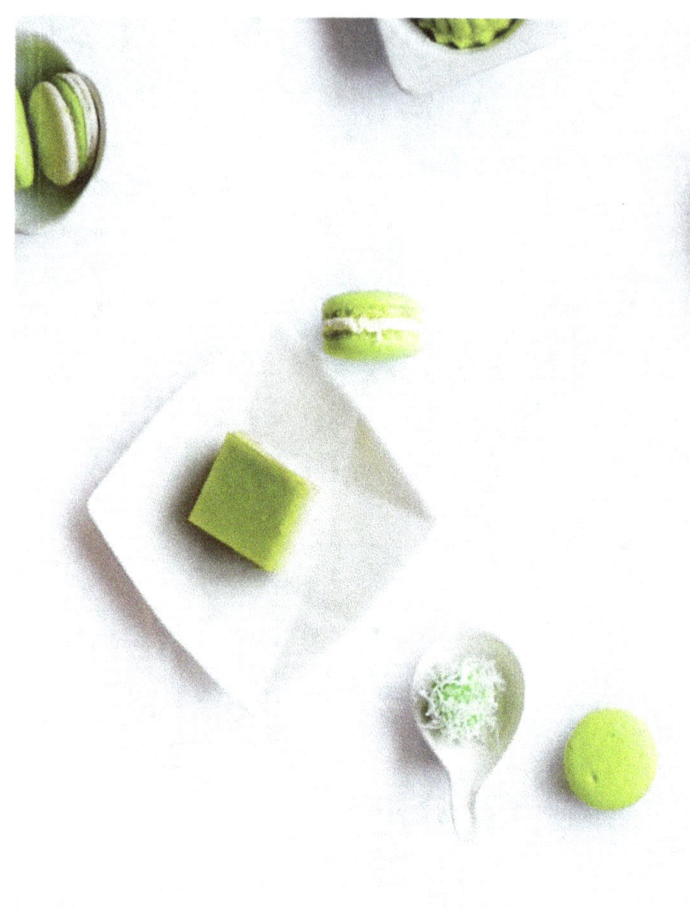

Use moringa as a flavouring for just about any dessert and cake. It's also a great colouring alternative to *pandan* when making Malaysian *kuih-muih* (traditional cakes): Boil fresh moringa leaves and add to the blender with a bit of water. You'll get a dark green paste that, when baked, results in a natural shade of green.

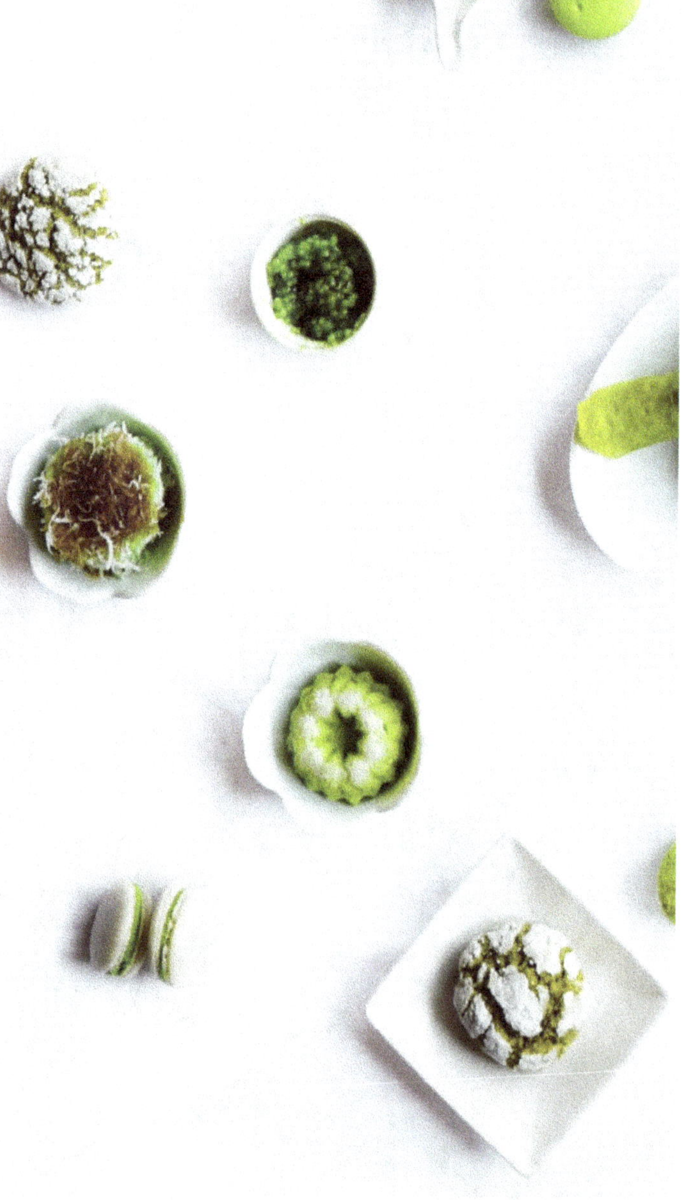

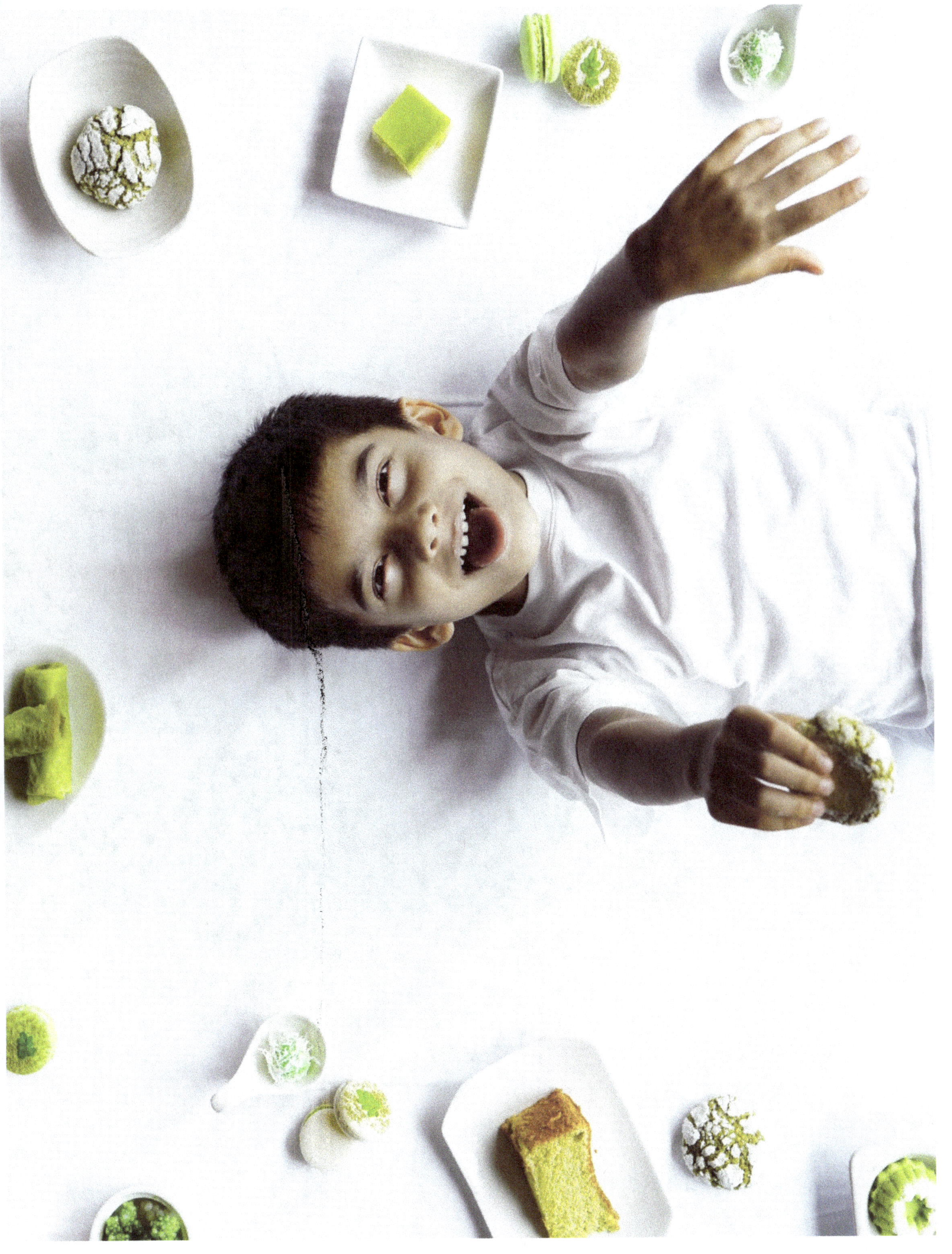

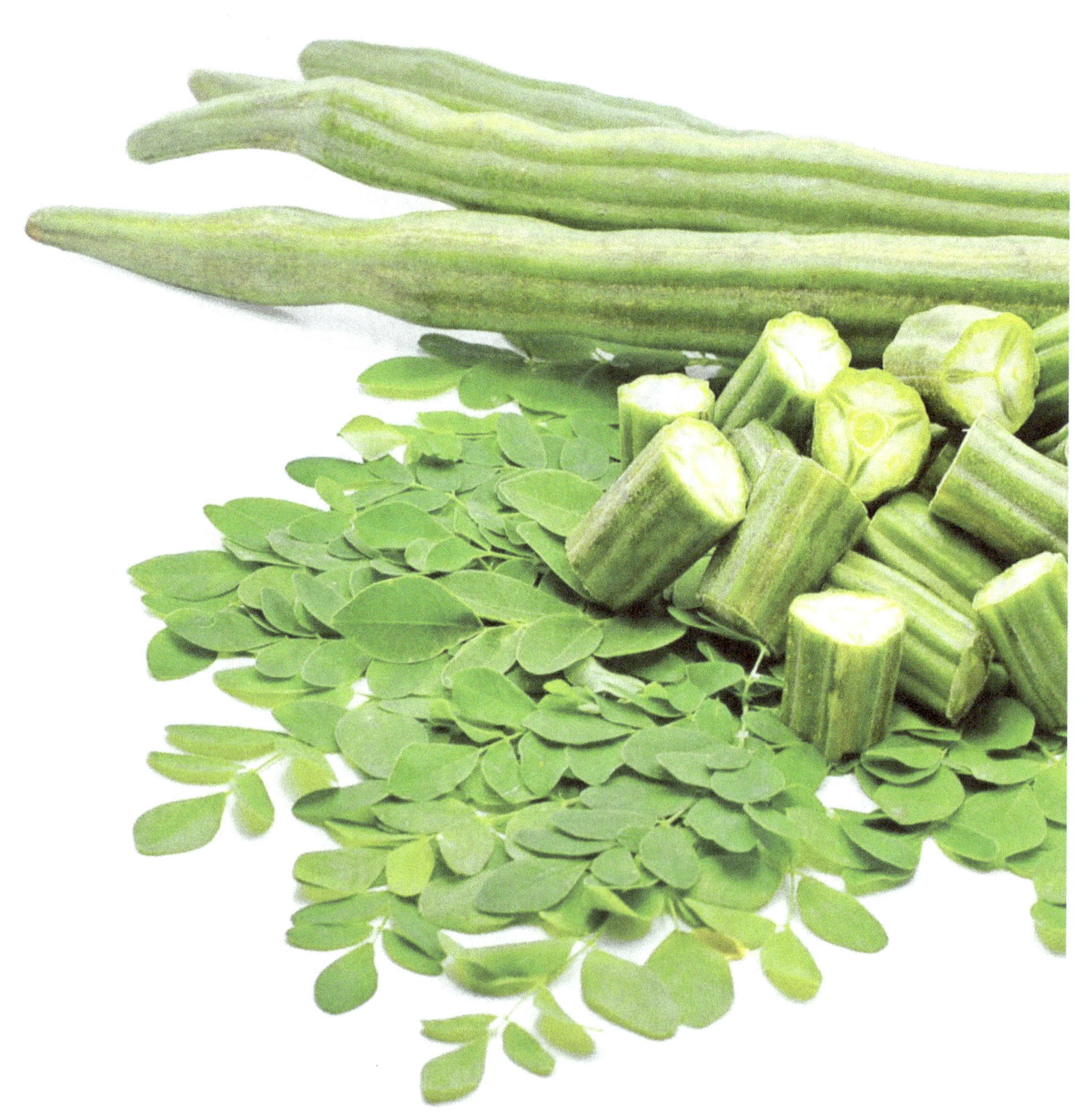

MORINGA DRUMSTICKS

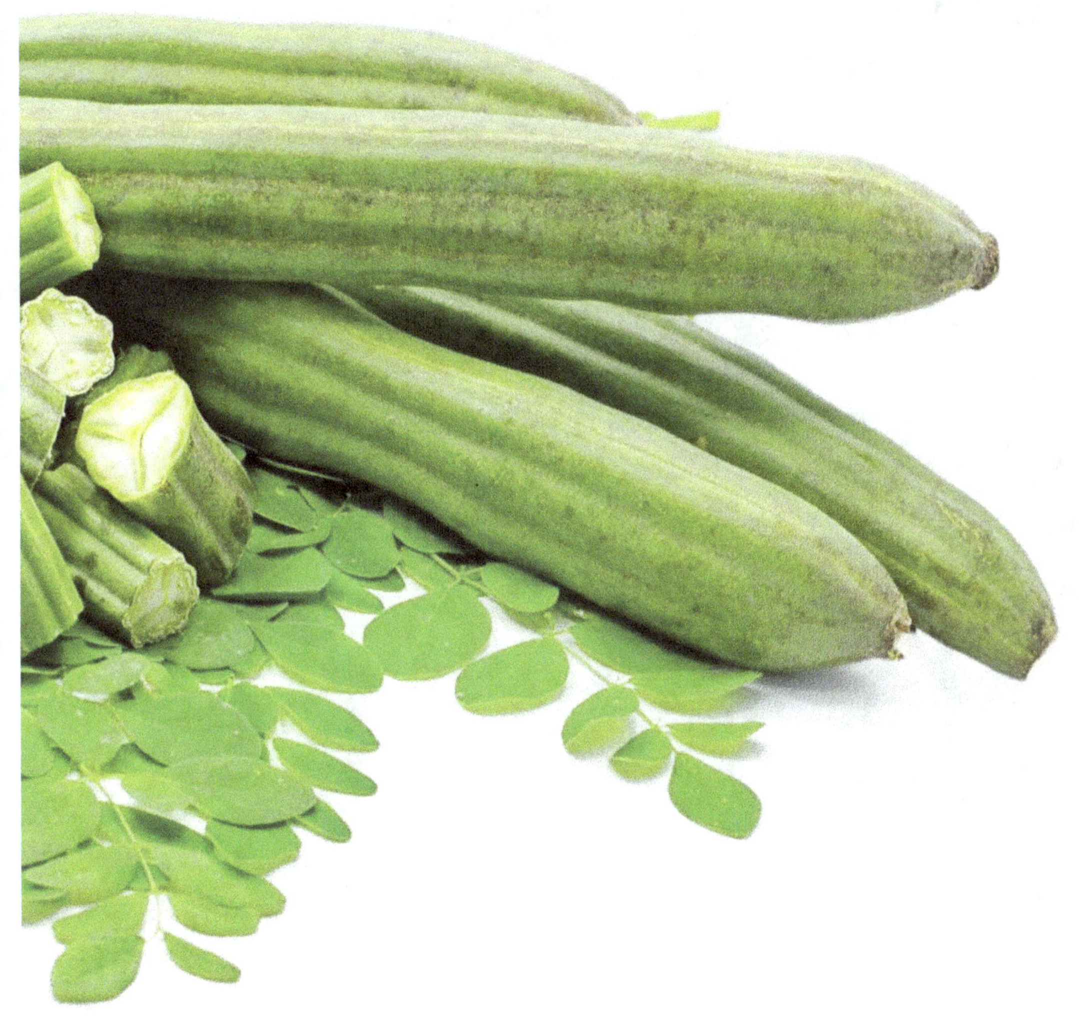

5 THINGS TO KNOW ABOUT DRUMSTICKS AND SEEDS

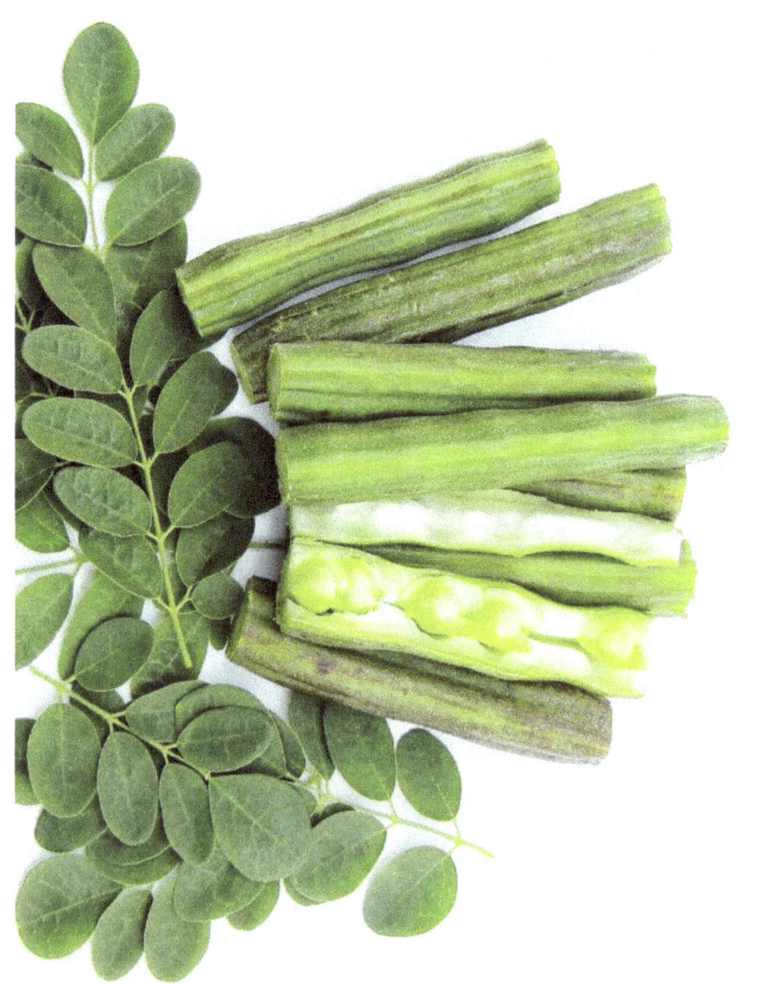

Drumsticks are the seed pods of the moringa tree and can be consumed as a vegetable. In India, it is prepared in a multitude of ways, paired with common ingredients that are found in most home kitchens.

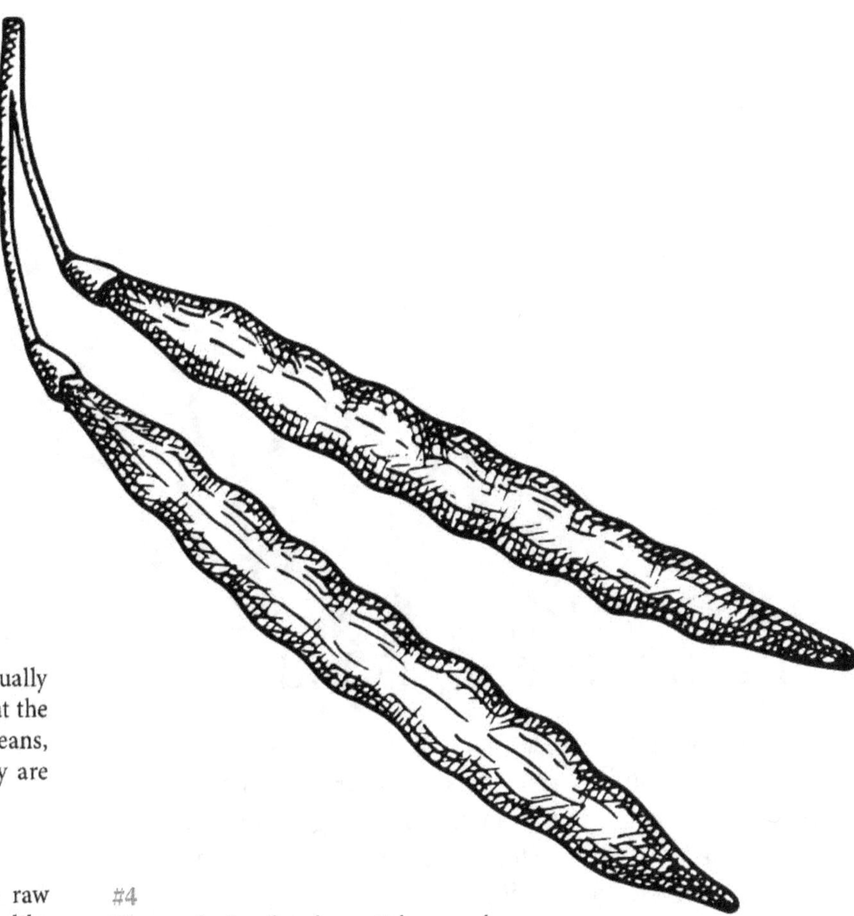

#1

When they are very young (usually about 12cm-20cm long), you can eat the drumsticks as you would green beans, edamame, or fresh garbanzo. They are sweet, crisp, and very delicious.

#2

Young drumsticks can be eaten raw right off the trees, or cooked just like any other vegetable. They can be added to salads or chopped into little pieces and added to stews, soups, casseroles, and sauces. You can also dry them and ground into powder, then add them to breads, muffins, or corn bread.

#3

When they get larger, the drumsticks tend to have a stringy texture and require longer cooking time. The older pods often taste like asparagus and can be substituted for that vegetable in recipes. Older drumsticks are often quite fibrous and hard to chew. Cut through the skin and eat the soft, gelatinous flesh inside.

#4

The seeds in the drumsticks can be popped like popcorn. They taste sweet at first and sometimes turn bitter in the mouth. They are rich in vitamins and minerals and are very, very potent for the body so go slow. Start with just a few seeds and let your system get accustomed to it.

#5

Moringa seeds have a superpower all their own: they can be used to separate unwanted particles, impurities, and sediment from water. These 'wastes' will then settle to the bottom of the water container and can be removed through filtration.

Ginataang Kalabasa

This Filipino vegetable stew dish traditionally features kabocha squash and coconut milk, as reflected in its name—*ginataang* is a Filipino word meaning "cooked with coconut milk" whereas *kalabasa* is a type of squash. In this version, I swapped squash for pumpkin and added moringa drumsticks to make it even more interesting.

Ingredients
2 pumpkin, cut into small peices
1 ½ cup coconut milk
2 tbsp cooking oil
3-4 moringa drumsticks, cut into 2- to 3-inch pieces
4 cloves garlic, minced
1 medium onion, chopped
1 thumb-sized ginger, cut into small pieces
Salt and pepper to taste
½ cup water as required

Method
1. Add oil to a pot over medium heat.
2. When the oil is hot, add chopped garlic and onion.
3. Stir until the aromatics turn translucent.
4. Add the ginger and pumpkin, and cook for a few minutes.
5. If the mixture seems dry at this point, add a bit of water.
6. Allow to simmer for 5-10 minutes, or until the pumpkin becomes soft.
7. Pour in the coconut milk.
8. Add the moringa drumsticks.
9. Gently stir and cook until the drumsticks are cooked.
10. Serve hot with steamed rice.

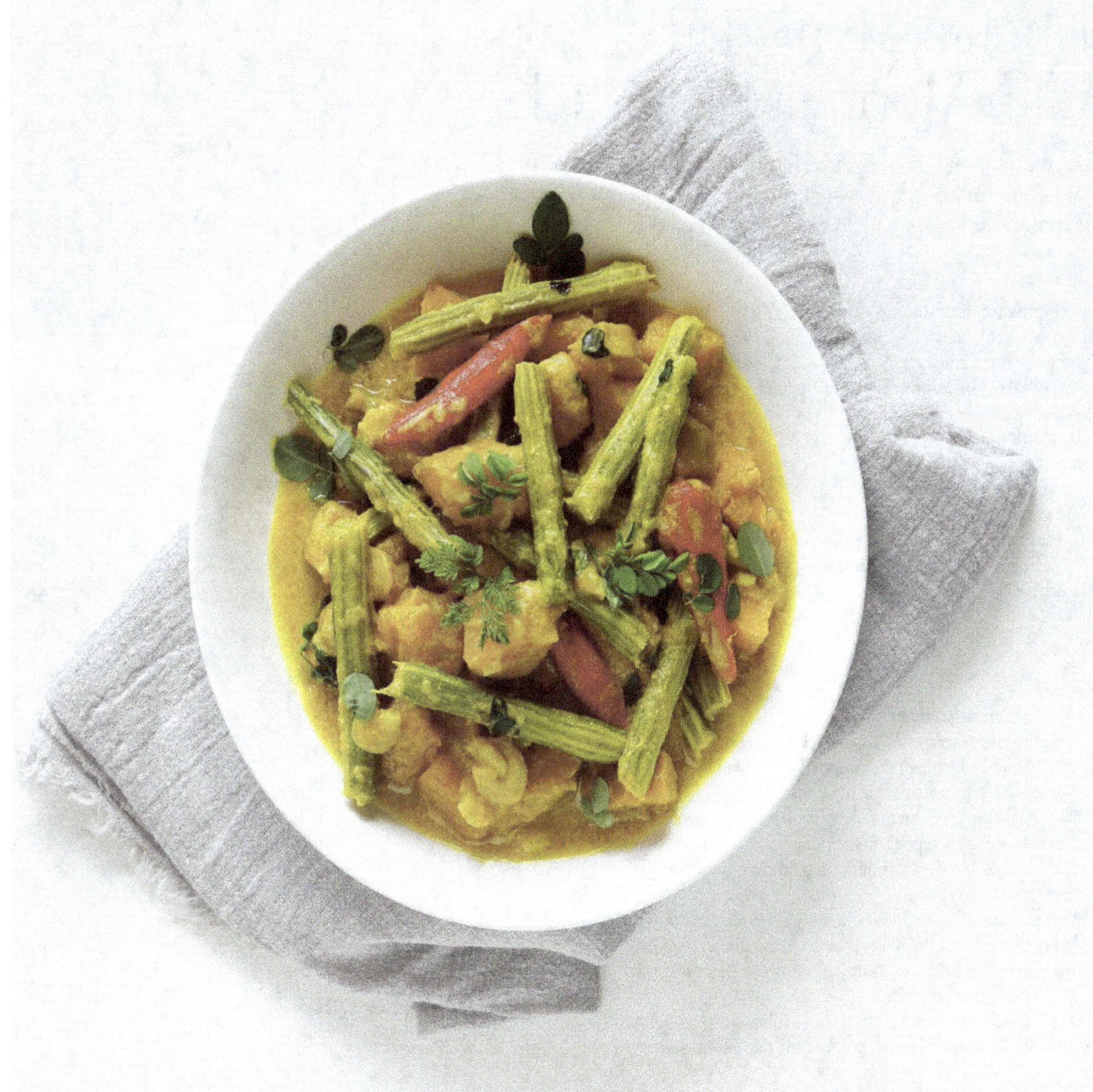

Tibetan Momo Dumplings With Moringa Drumsticks

The unofficial national dish of Tibet is a highly adaptable dish that can be made vegan, vegetarian, or with meat. We added the flesh of moringa drumsticks to take this recipe to another level.

Ingredients (makes about 6 dumplings)
2-inch knob of fresh ginger, peeled and chopped coarsely
3 garlic cloves, crushed
14gm shiitake mushroom, soaked in 1 cup of boiling water
2 cups spinach, chopped
2 green onions, chopped
¼ cup chopped coriander leaves
1 ½ kg firm tofu
¼ cup grated carrots
2 tbsp soy sauce
2-3 moringa drumsticks, cut into 2-inch peices
Steamer basket
1 packet of dumpling wrappers

Method
1. Boil the drumsticks with a little salt.
2. When cooked, scrape the drumstick flesh with a spoon.
3. Place in a bowl with all the chopped ingredients.
4. Season with soy sauce, salt and pepper.
5. Mix everything together.
6. Lay a dumpling wrapper on the palm of your hand.
7. Scoop a small heap of the dumpling mixture onto the centre of the wrapper.
8. Using your thumb and index finger of the other hand, bring the edges of the wrapper around the filling, pleating the wrapper at intervals while gathering the edges together at the top. Pinch to seal.
9. Repeat with remaining wrappers and fillings.
10. Transfer to steamer basket, keeping the dumplings ½-inch apart.
11. Cover the basket with a tight-fitting lid or aluminium foil and steam for about 10-12 minutes on high heat.
12. Transfer to a plate and cover with aluminium foil to keep warm until ready to serve.
13. Serve with dipping sauce of your choice.

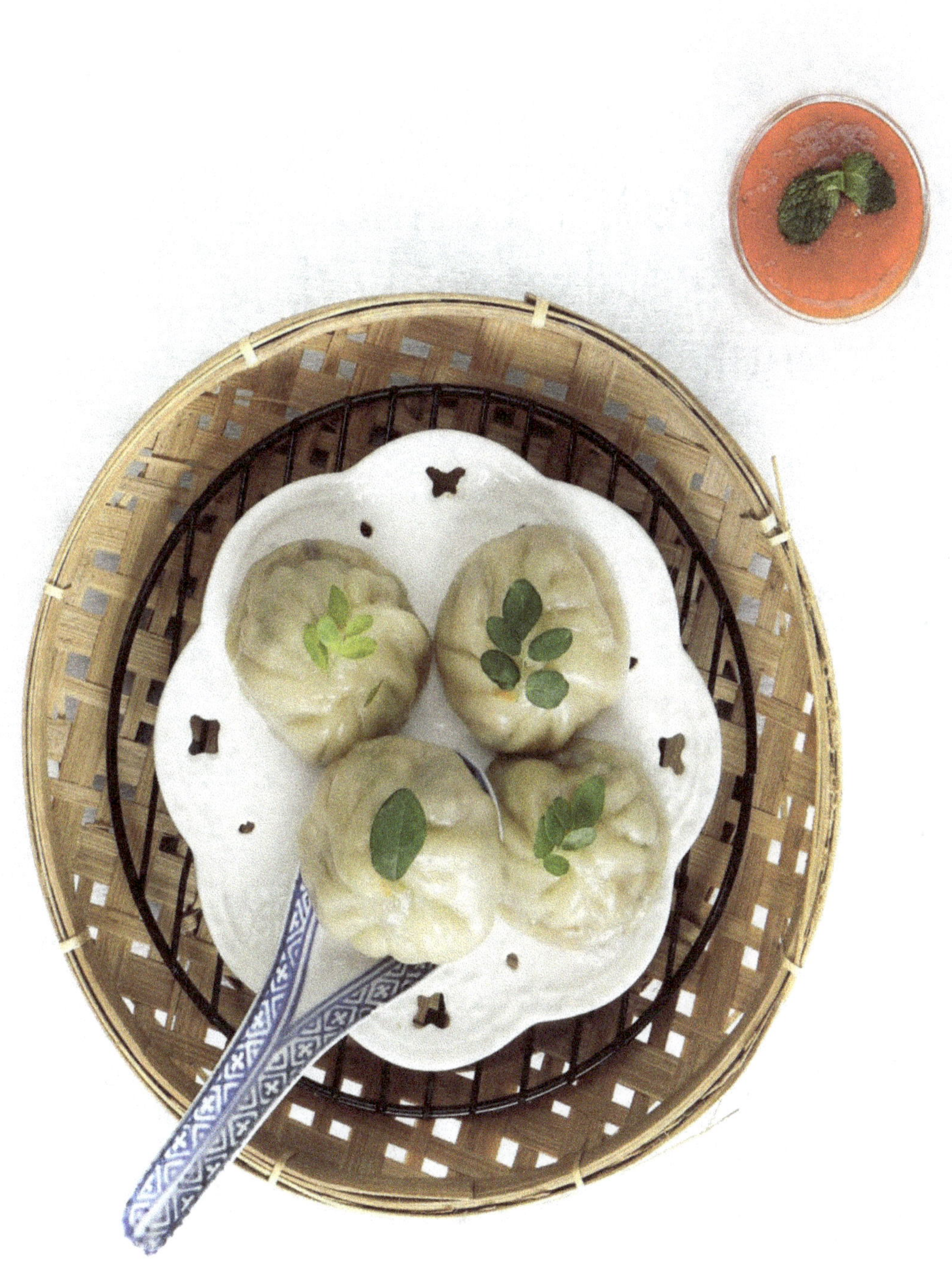

Persian-Style Sweet And Spicy Drumsticks Cooked In Coconut Water

The addition of fresh coconut water balances out the spiciness while adding a natural sweetness to this dish.

Ingredients
2 moringa drumsticks
300ml fresh coconut water

To grind
3 green chillies
½ cup fresh coriander leaves, finely chopped
1 inch ginger
4 cloves
3 tbsp fresh coconut flesh
1 tsp turmeric powder
Salt to taste
2 tbsp ghee for cooking

Method
1. Peel the drumsticks and cut into 1- to 2-inch sticks.
2. Heat up a pan.
3. Fry all the spices meant for grinding.
4. Let cool, and grind into a smooth paste.
5. Heat ghee in a pan.
6. Sauté the drumsticks for a few minutes.
7. Add the ground spices.
8. Add the coconut water and simmer for about 15-20 minutes.
9. Serve hot with rice.

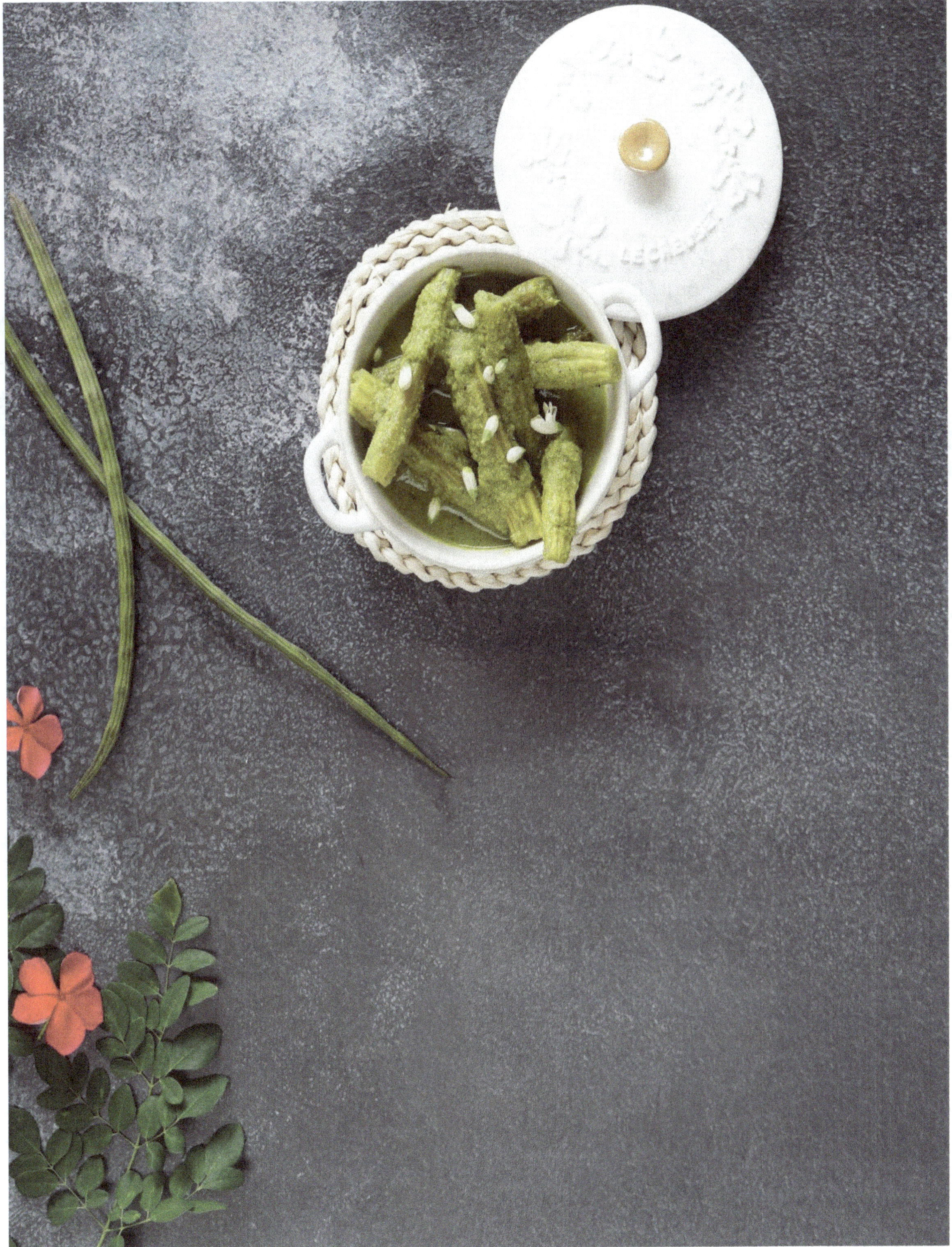

Mutton With Moringa Drumsticks

Tender, fall-off-the-bone mutton pairs so well with the soft flesh of the moringa drumsticks in this moreish dish.

Ingredients

5-6 drumsticks, scraped and cut into 2- to 3-inch sticks
500gm mutton
5 tbsp oil
2 onions, finely chopped
1 tbsp ginger-garlic paste
2-3 tomato, finely chopped
2 tsp red chilli powder
2 tsp coriander powder
2 tsp cumin powder
1 tsp turmeric powder
2 tsp garam masala
Salt to taste
Fresh coriander leaves (for garnishing)

Method

1. Heat oil in a pressure cooker if available, or in a regular pot.
2. Fry the onions till translucent.
3. Add the mutton pieces and ginger-garlic paste.
4. Cook till all the water dries up
5. Add the tomatoes, red chilli powder, coriander powder, turmeric powder, and cumin powder.
6. Add salt and mix well.
7. Pour in one cup of water.
8. Close the lid and cook for 3 to 4 whistles or until the meat is cooked
9. Open the lid of the pressure cooker. Check that the mutton is cooked through and the oil is separated from the curry.
10. Add the moringa drumsticks.
11. Cook for about 10-12 minutes, or until the drumstick is cooked through.
12. Add garam masala.
13. Simmer for another 10 minutes.
14. Garnish with fresh coriander leaves and serve with rice or roti.

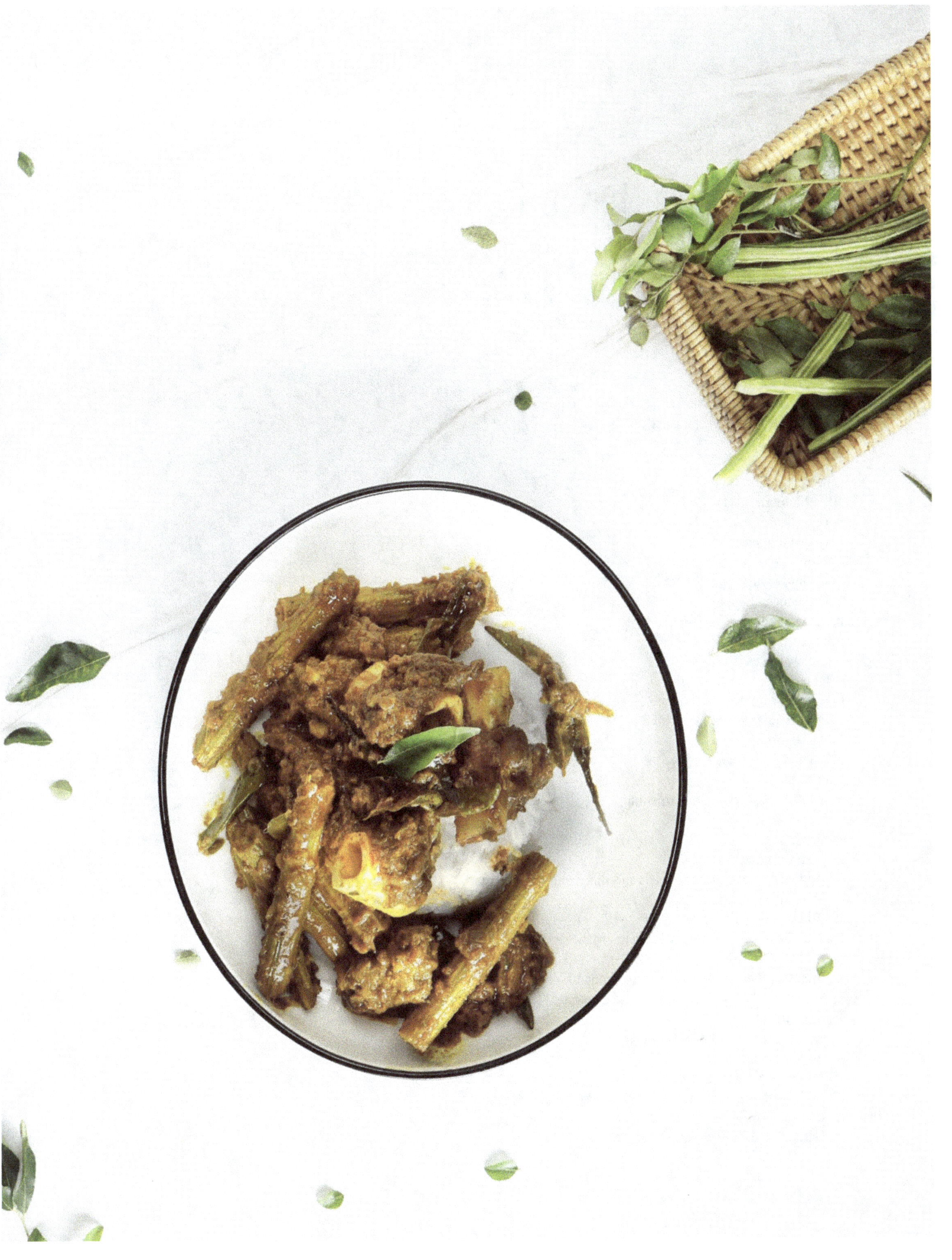

Drumstick Biryani

Biryani is a mixed rice dish that can be traced to the
Muslims of South Asia. It is made with Indian spices,
vegetables, rice, and usually some kind of meat. This
unique version uses moringa drumsticks.

Ingredients

2 cups basmati rice, washed and soaked for 30 minutes
3-4 moringa drumsticks, washed and peeled,
then cut into 2-inch sticks
3 tbsp ghee
1 inch cinnamon stick
4-5 cardamom pods
5-6 cloves
1 tsp cumin seeds
2 onions, sliced
2 tsp ginger-garlic paste
2-3 tomatoes, chopped
1 tbsp chili powder
1 tbsp coriander powder
A few bay leaves
2 star anise
1 cup fresh mint leaves, chopped
1 cup coriander leaves, chopped
2 tbsp yogurt
1 tbsp biryani masala
4 cups water
A handful of cashews (for garnishing)

Method

1. Heat the ghee in a pot.
2. Add whole spices, cumin seeds and sliced onions. Sauté for
    about five minutes.
3. Add ginger-garlic paste and mix well
4. Add the moringa drumsticks, followed by tomatoes.
5. Add chilli powder, turmeric powder, and salt.
6. Mix well, then cover and cook for about 10 minutes.
7. Stir in the chopped mint leaves and coriander leaves.
8. Add yogurt.
9. Cover and cook for a few minutes.
10. Add biryani masala.
11. Add soaked basmati rice.
12. Add water, mix well, and cook till the rice is done. This should
    take 15-20 minutes.
13. Garnish with cashews and serve hot.

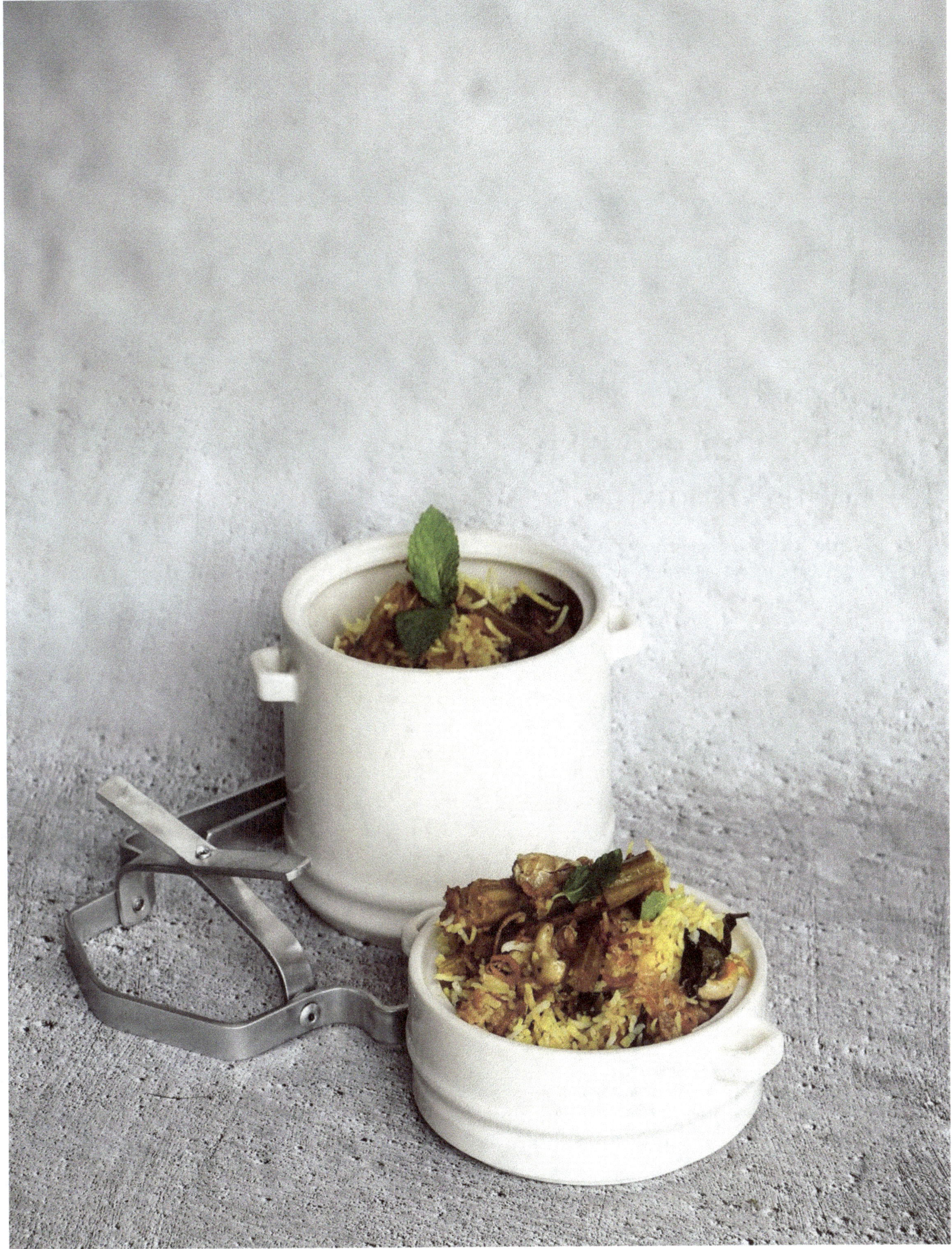

Myanmarese Fish Curry With Drumsticks

Tangy, spicy and so satisfying when eaten with steamed white rice or your favourite roti.

Ingredients
3-4 fish fillet of your choice
8-10 pieces of moringa drumsticks
1 medium-sized onion, finely minced
3-4 cloves garlic, finely minced
1-inch knob of ginger, minced
2-3 ripe tomatoes, quartered
½ tsp turmeric powder
½ tsp chilli powder
2 tbsp fish sauce
2-3 tbsp oil
1 tsp fresh tamarind flesh, rinsed and mashed
Coriander for garnishing

Method
1. Cut fish into desired size.
2. Wash, cut and rinse the moringa drumsticks.
3. Heat oil in a pan.
4. Add onions, ginger, and garlic. Stir for a few minutes.
5. Add chopped tomatoes, chilli powder, and turmeric powder.
6. Stir for 1-2 minutes.
7. Add fish and moringa drumsticks.
8. Add water and let simmer on low heat for 10-15 minutes.
9. Add tamarind and simmer for a few more minutes.
10. Add fish sauce. Garnish with coriander leaves to serve.

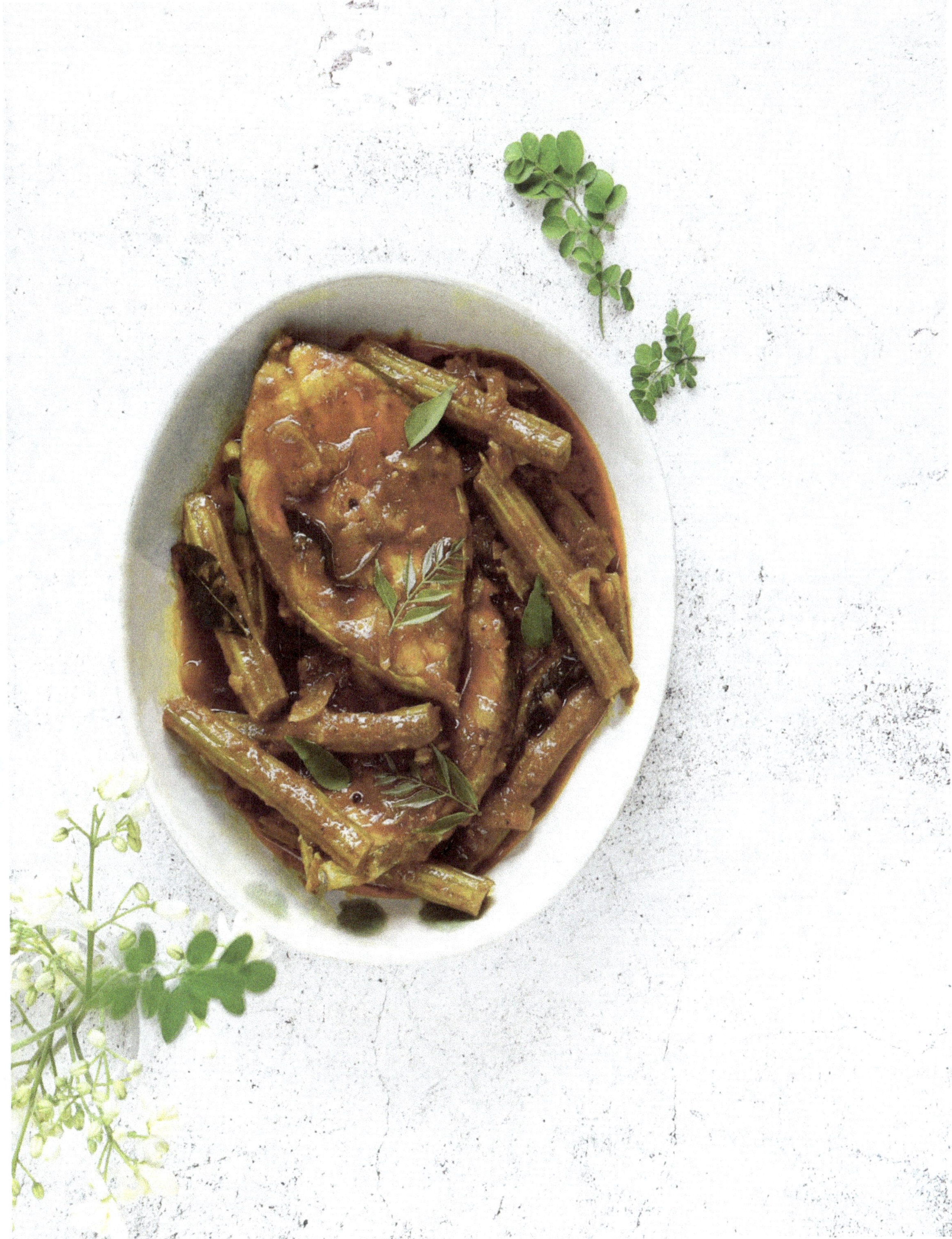

Drumstick With Potatoes

The simple yet satisfying combination of potatoes and
moringa drumsticks is comfort food at its best.

Ingredients
3-4 drumsticks (cut into finger-length sticks)
2-3 medium potatoes, diced
3-4 medium onions, finely chopped
2-3 medium tomatoes, finely chopped
1-2 green chillies, halved length-wise
½ tsp red chilli powder
½ tsp cumin seeds
½ tsp mustard seeds
¼ tsp turmeric powder
1 tsp coriander powder
½ tsp chilli powder
½ tbsp garam masala
2 tbsp oil
1 stalk curry leaves
2-3 tbsp fresh coriander leaves, chopped

Method
1. Peel and cut potatoes. Place in a bowl of water until ready to use.
2. In a pan, add 2 tbsp oil.
3. Add mustard seeds and cumin seeds.
4. When they splutter, add curry leaves.
5. Add split green chillies and onions. Fry until onions become transparent.
6. Add drumsticks and potatoes. Fry for 2-3 minutes.
7. Add chopped tomatoes.
8. Add turmeric powder and salt to taste.
9. Fry until tomatoes turn mushy.
10. Add red chilli powder, coriander powder, and garam masala.
11. Pour enough water to cover drumstick and potatoes.
12. Cover and cook until the vegetables are cooked through.
13. Garnish with coriander leaves.
14. Serve hot with rice or roti.

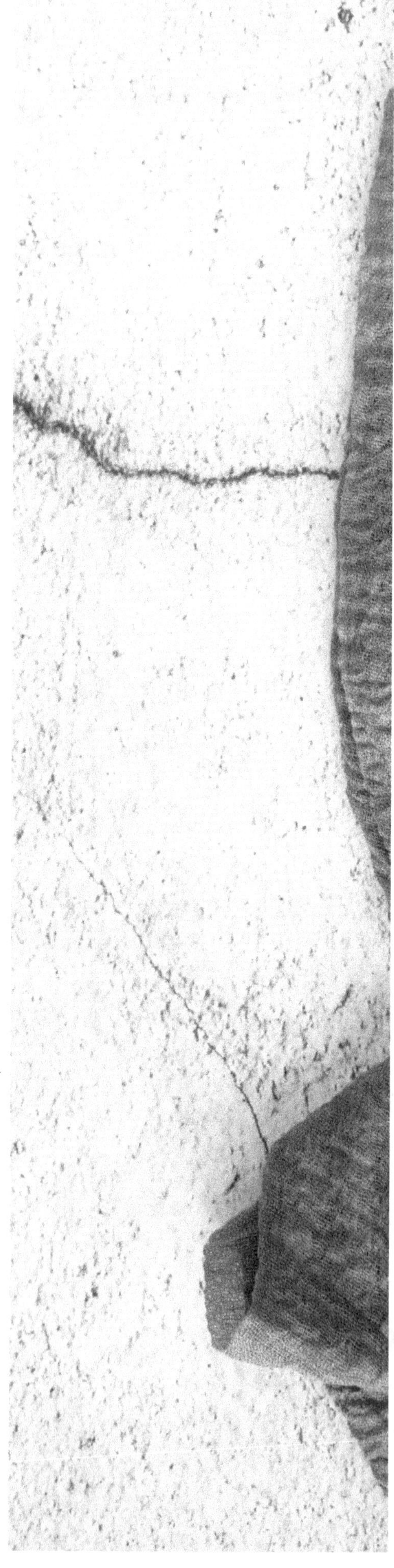

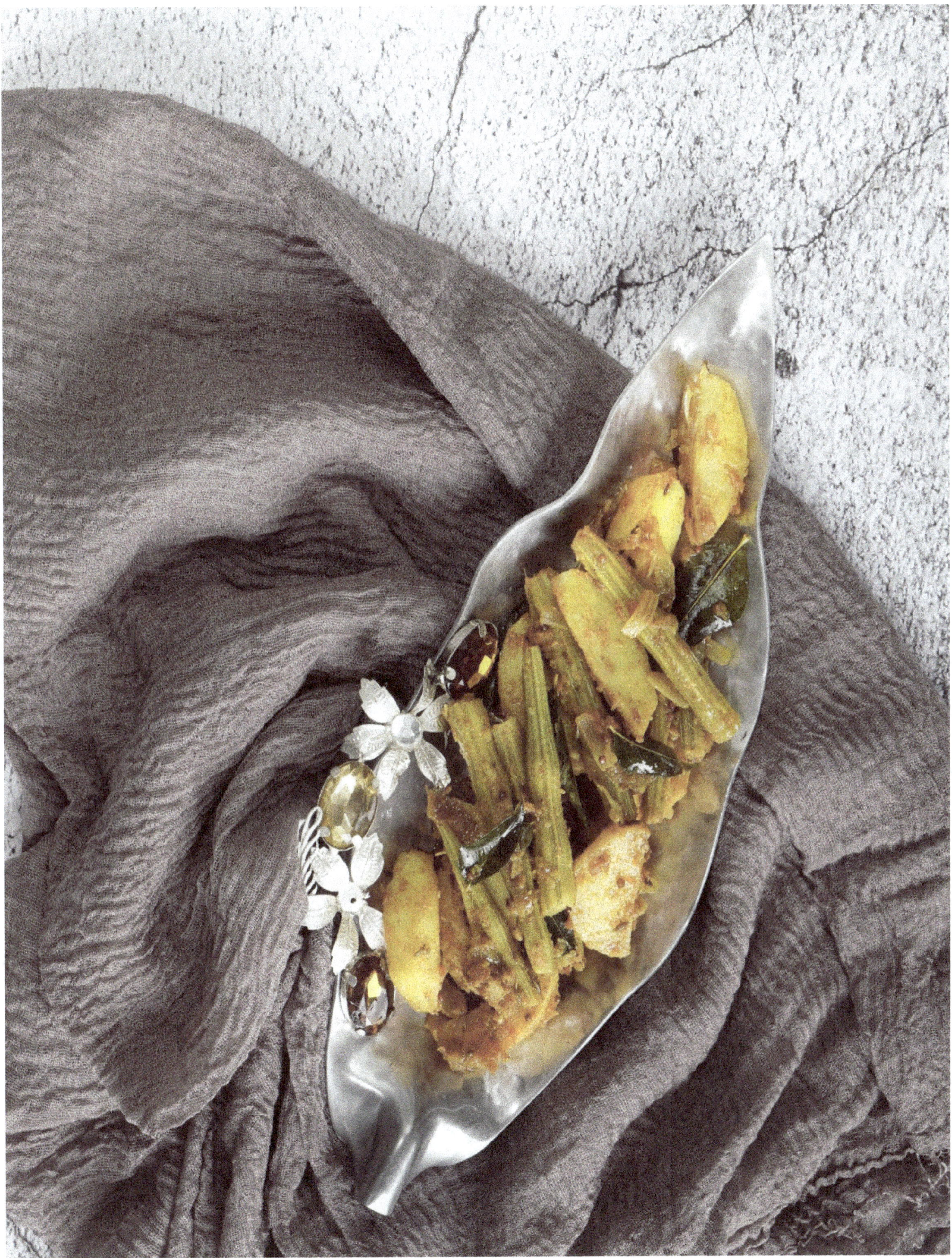

Toor Dal With Drumsticks

Growing up in Myanmar, one of my earliest recollections about food was the smell of *dal* cooking in the kitchen. In those days, food was cooked with charcoal or fire wood. It took a long time for the *dal* to cook so we would start first thing in the morning. I would wake up to the aroma of cooking *dal* permeating the house. We almost always cooked this dish with fresh moringa drumsticks. Till now, each time I make this *dal*, it brings back such beautiful childhood memories.

Ingredients
1 1/2 cup *toor dal*
1 1/2 tsp cumin seeds
1 tsp mustard seeds
3-4 cloves of garlic, chopped
2 big onion, chopped
3 tsp chopped ginger
¾ tsp turmeric powder
1 tsp chilli powder
1 tsp coriander powder
1 tsp cumin powder
Pinch of *asefoetida*
2-3 green chillies, chopped
2-4 tomatoes, chopped
2-3 drumsticks
2-3 tbsp ghee
A few curry leaves
Fresh coriander leaves for garnishing (optional)
Salt to taste

Method
1. Wash, then soak the *dal* for at least one hour.
2. Cut the moringa drumsticks into 2- to 3-inch pieces.
3. Transfer the *dal* to a pressure cooker (you can also cook in a regular pot on the stove top but it will take longer).
4. Add water, ginger, garlic, tomatoes, turmeric powder, cumin powder, coriander powder, chilli powder, and the moringa drumsticks.
5. Pressure cook till about 4 whistles or all the ingredients are cooked.
6. Heat ghee in a pan and temper the mustard seeds and cumin seeds.
7. Add *asofoetida*, chopped onions, and curry leaves.
8. Pour this tempered ingredients into the *dal*.
9. Garnish with chopped coriander leaves to serve.

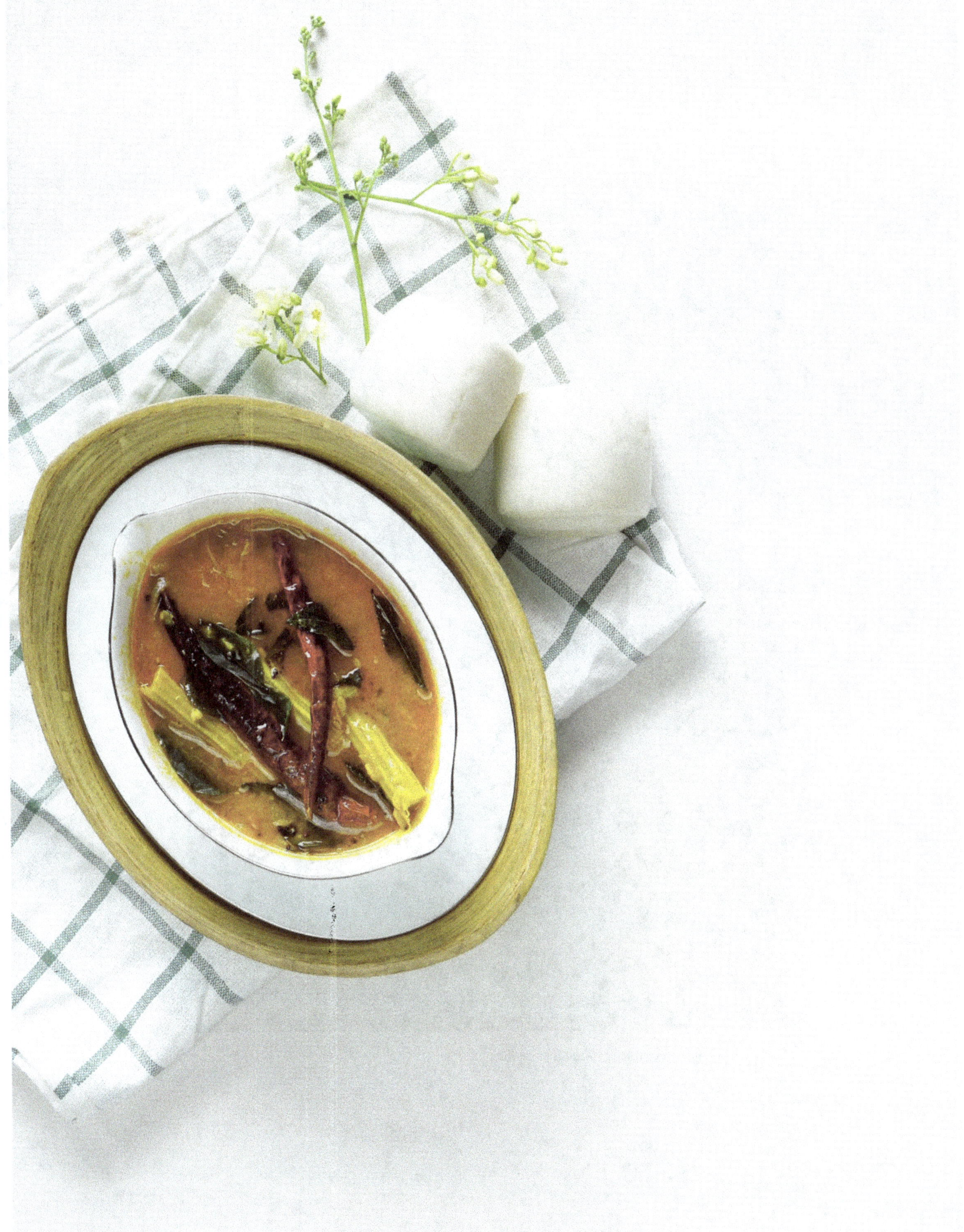

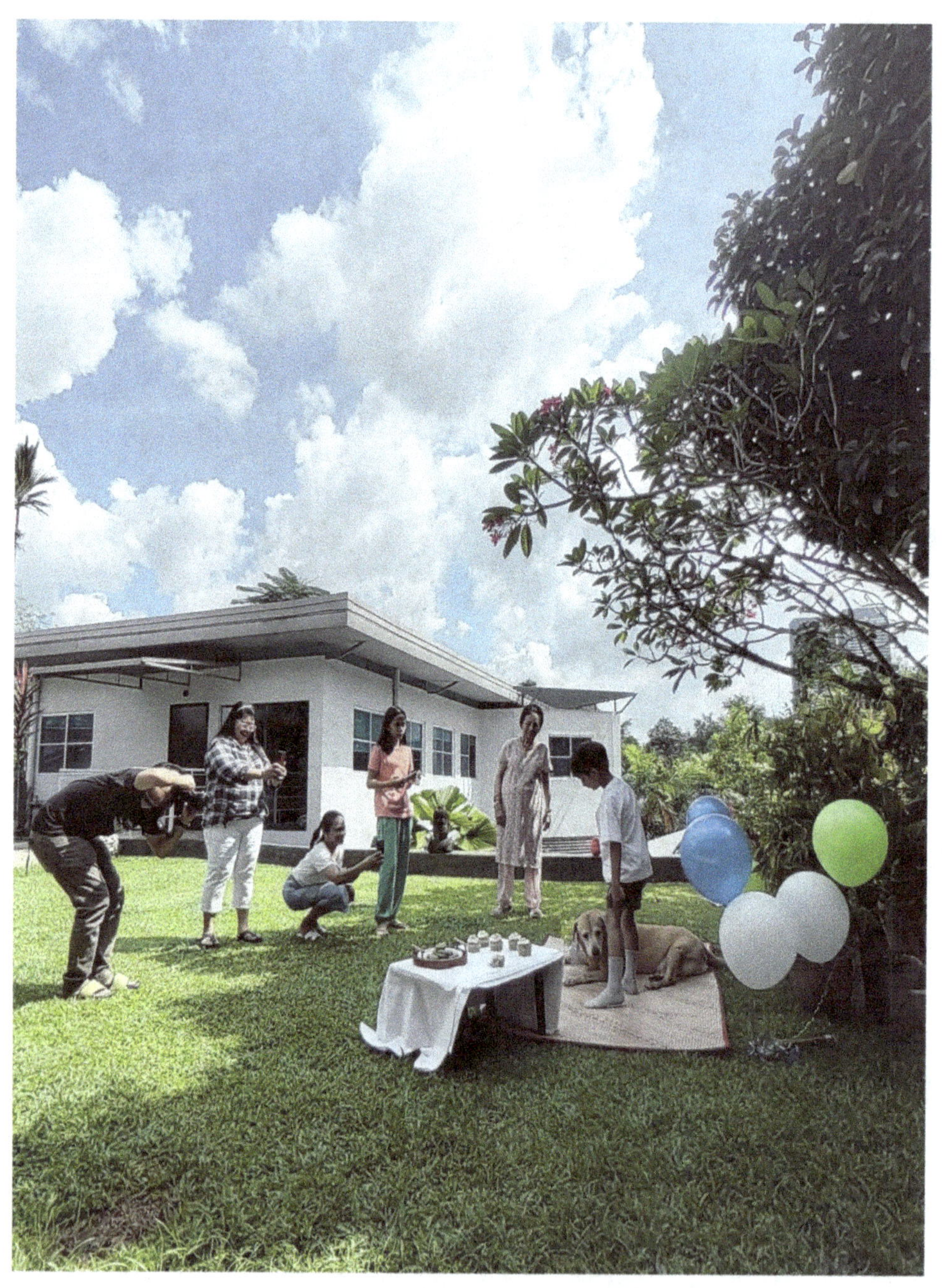

How many people does it take to shoot one photo?

The Making of *Moringalicious*

The photoshoot for *Moringalicious* took place over nearly three months and was held at Mohana's home, where every dish was made from scratch and prepared freshly using moringa leaves, flowers, and drumsticks from her garden. The whole process was laborious and creative, and involved just about everyone at home—including Mohana's beloved grandson, Ari, and their pets!

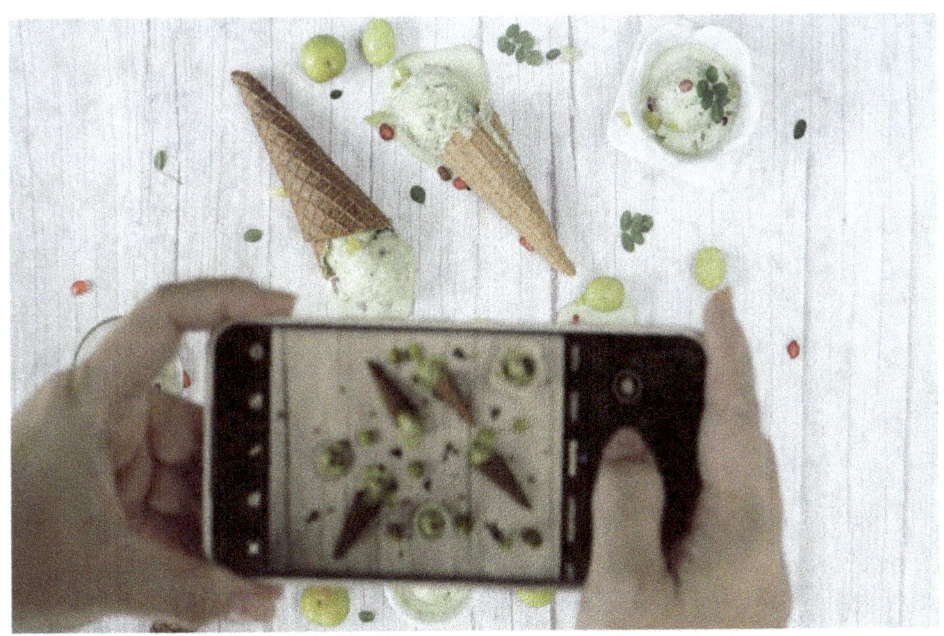

No ice-cream was harmed for this shot, though some of it melted

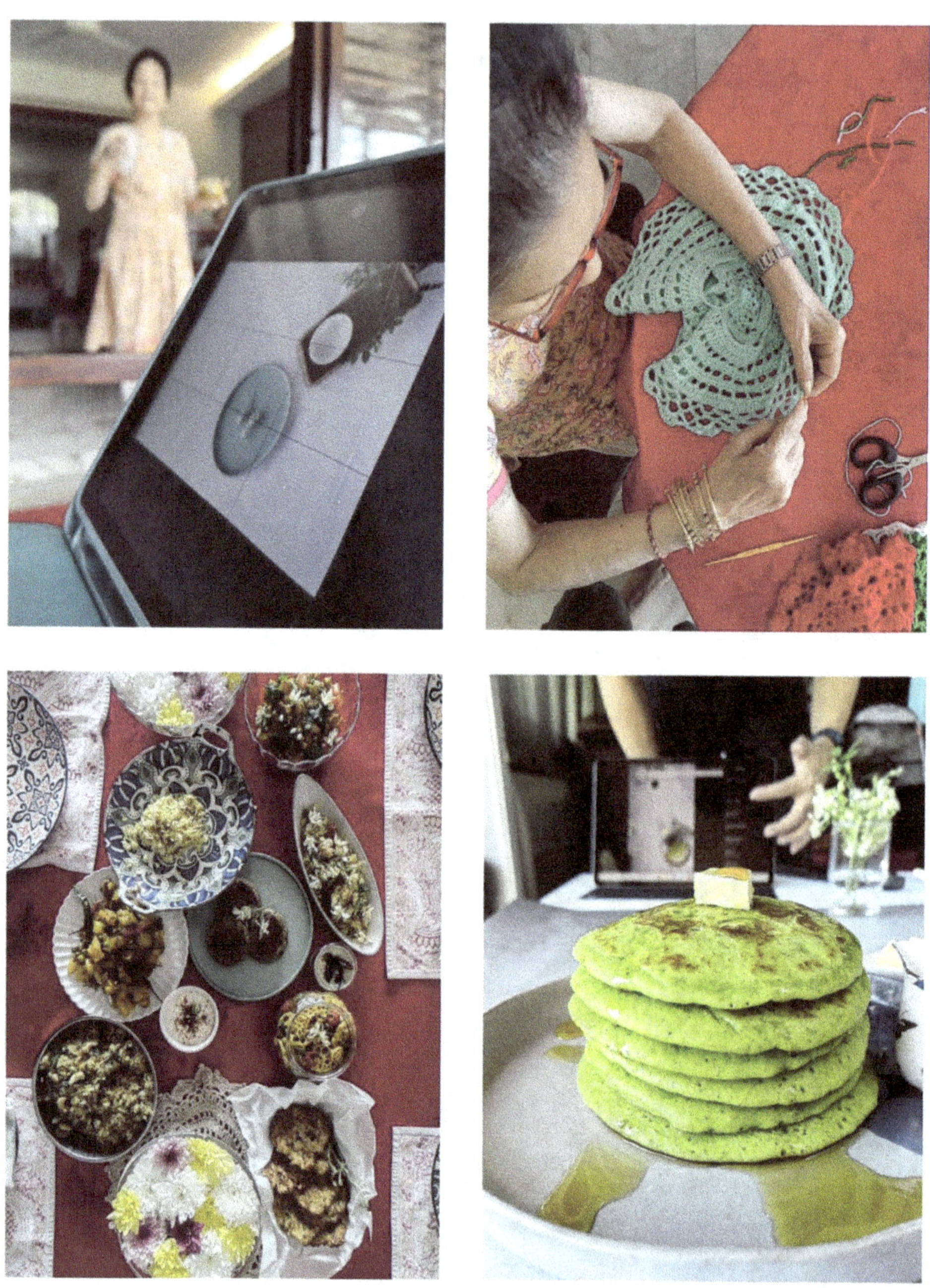

Clockwise from top left: Image check every step of the way; Mohana crocheted a bunch of doilies, see if you can spot them in the recipe photos; the best pancake stack; another shoot day, another moringa feast

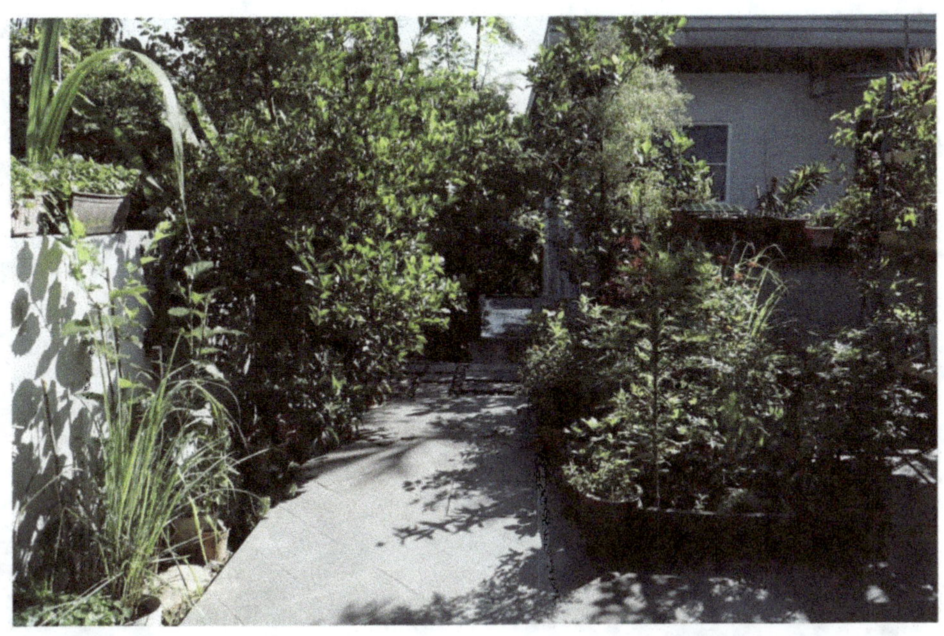

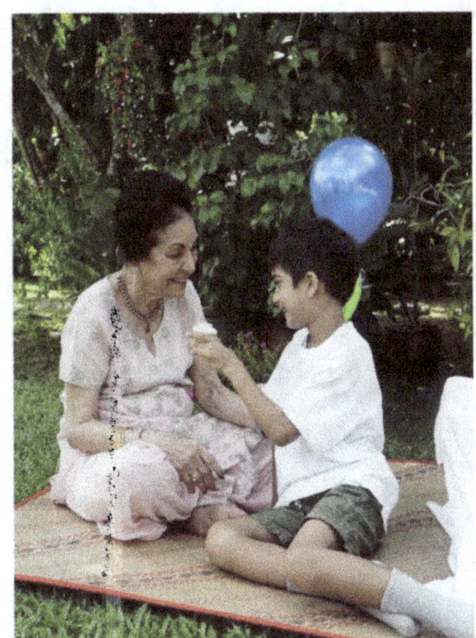

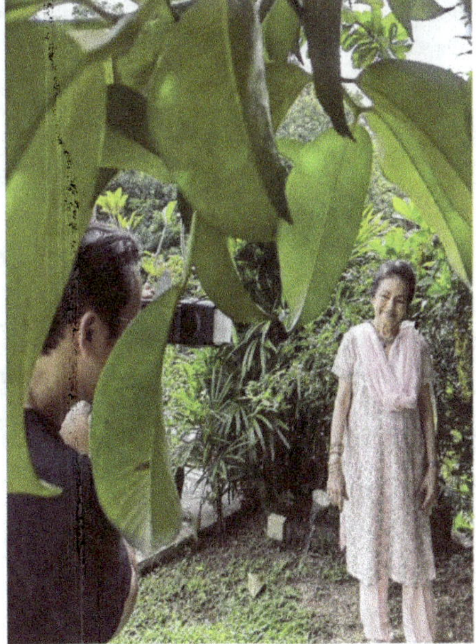

Clockwise from top: This herb patch is part of Mohana's garden; Mohana getting her portrait taken at her garden; a tender moment between Mohana and Ari

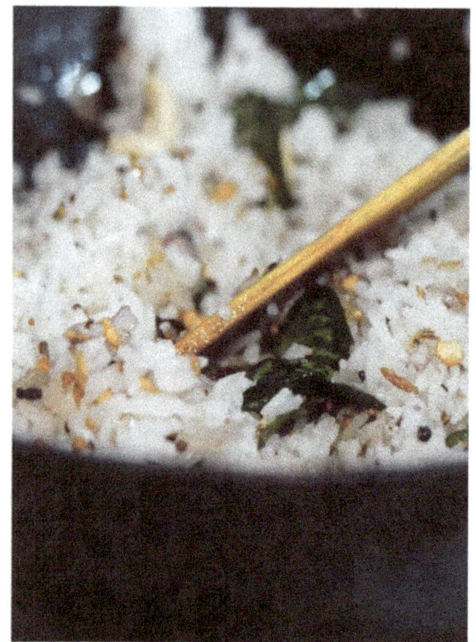

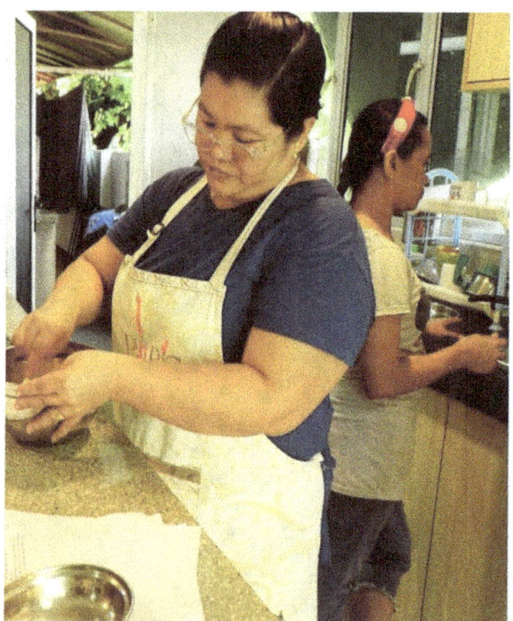

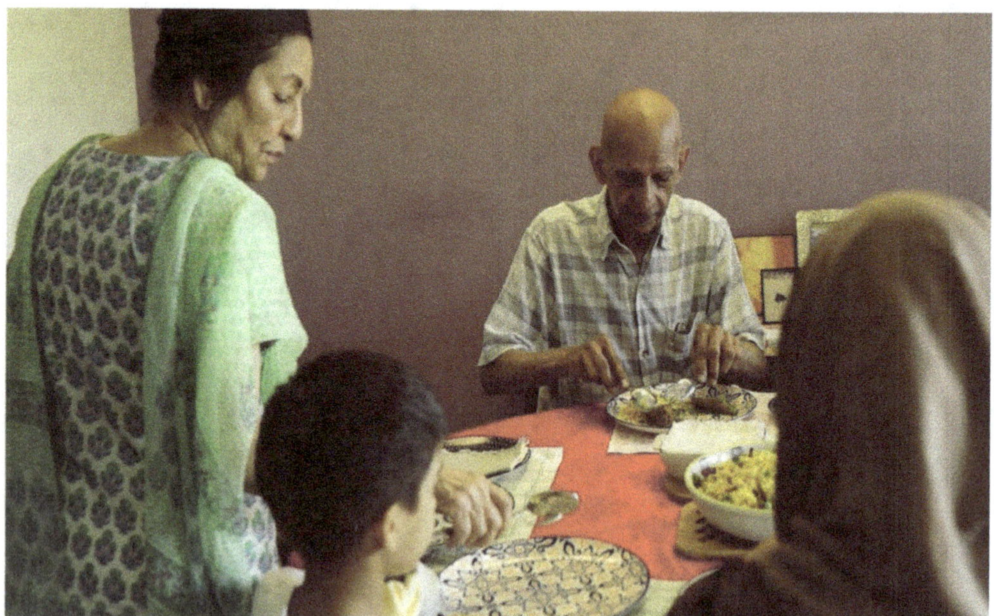

Clockwise from top left: The pulao was one of the top favourites among the team; Lyn and Christine helped prepare every dish from scratch; the team at lunch, tucking into the very dishes we shot earlier

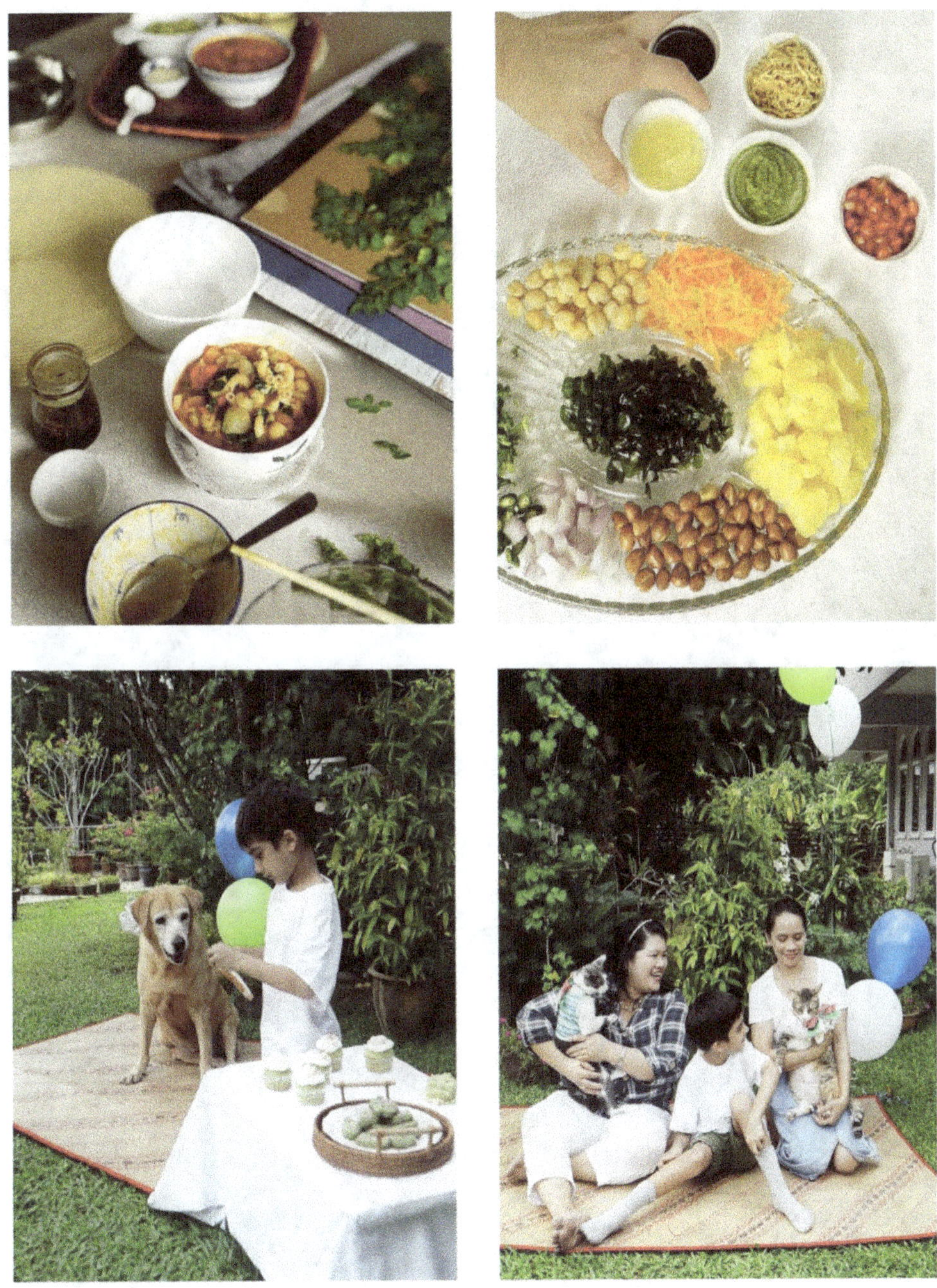

Clockwise from top left: Every dish goes from the kitchen to the plating table to be made camera-ready; shooting the Moringa Leaf Chaat; the one where nobody looks at the camera; here Mindy, you want some bread?

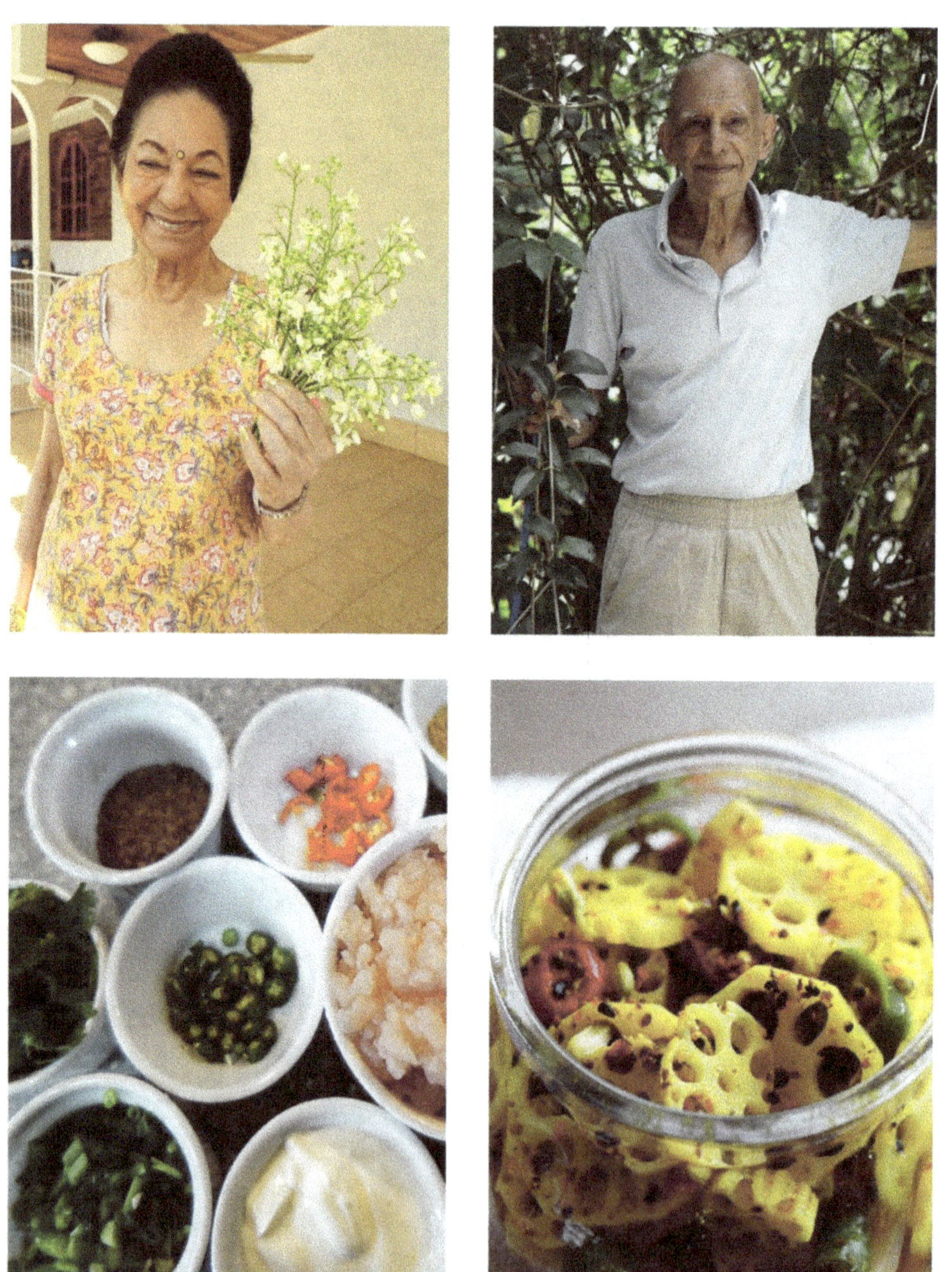

Clockwise from top left: Luckily for us, the moringa trees flowered in time for our photoshoot! Dr SS Gill, Mohana's husband; a close-up of the amazing moringa flower pickles; fresh ingredients ready to be whipped into yet another amazing dish

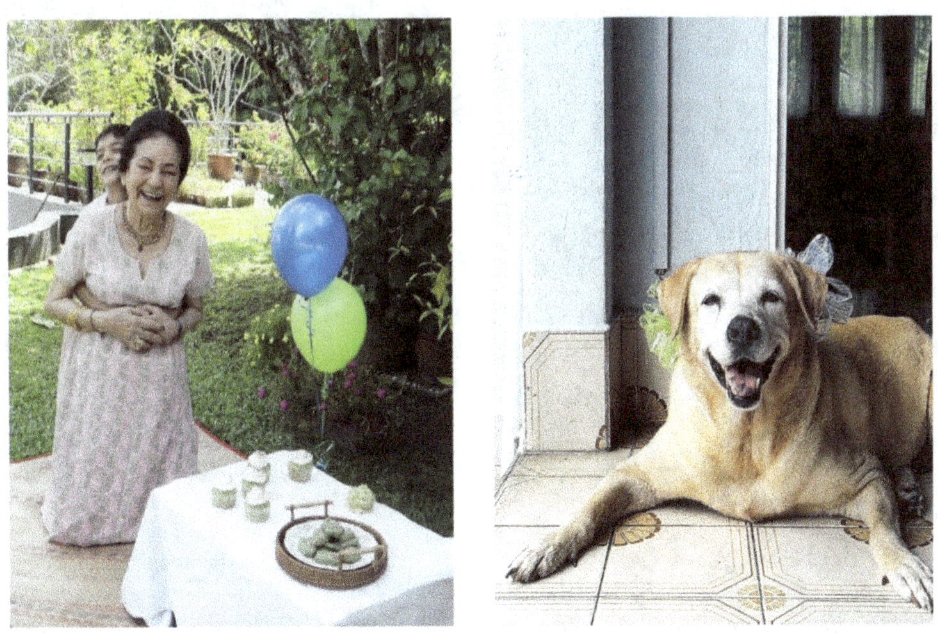

From left: Ari trying to lift Mohana up; aren't you the happiest girl at the shoot, Mindy?

About the Author

Mohana R Gill, or Rose Gill as she is affectionately known, was born in Burma, now called Myanmar. She has a Bachelor's degree from the University of Rangoon and an MBA from the University of Toronto. She was on the staff of the University of Rangoon till the military overthrew the Government in 1963, wherein she left for Malaysia. In 1965, she was an economics lecturer at the University of Malaya. Mohana retired when her first child was born, to focus on bringing up her children.

She travels extensively and maintains homes in Australia, India and the United States. Known amongst friends and relatives as the Travelling Gourmet, Mohana's deep love for cooking and her experimental approach in the kitchen is reflected in the way she mixes the old with the new, dishing up inventive and original recipes each time.

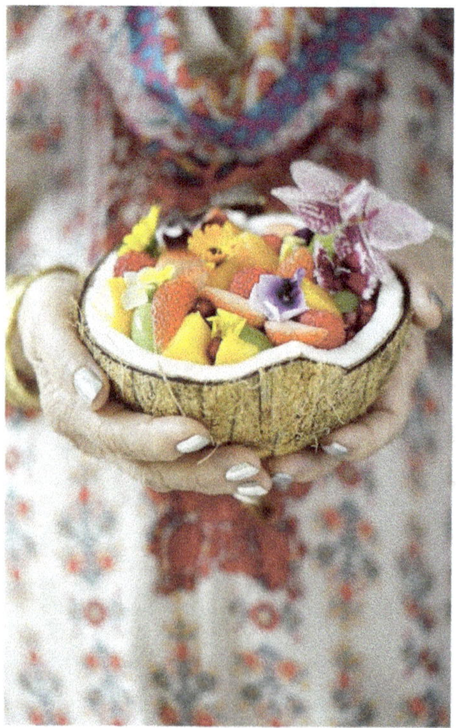

Fruitastic! was her first endeavour into the world of publishing and this was followed closely by *Vegemania!*. Both books were met with much critical acclaim and enthusiastic response, and went on to pick up coveted accolades at the Gourmand World Cookbook Awards, the Oscar-equivalent of the cookbook industry. Completing the series is *Flowerlicious*, which focuses on the benefits of edible flowers. *Flowerlicious* bagged the prestigious Gourmand World Cookbook Awards, for Best In All–Malaysia award, and was named Top 3 in the Natural Health Category in 2019. It was also a Finalist in the Book Excellence Awards 2019. To date, Mohana is the only Malaysian to have won eight 'Best in the World' awards.

In between all that, Mohana found time to author *Hayley's Happylicious*, a series of books that promotes good nutrition and wellbeing among children. The titular character is a squirrel that takes young readers on fun, food-filled adventures while exploring popular Asian folk tales and Malaysian legends. The series, as Mohana sees it, is Malaysia's gift to the world.

Mohana's most personal project to date is an eponymous biography about her beloved mother, Leela, that chronicles life in pre-war Burma and how she fought against the odds to bring up five children on her own. An intimate collection of memories and treasured moments, it captures the courage, determination, and perseverance that Leela was known for and traces her journey from her home country to America and the Canadian Rockies.

List of Awards

FRUITASTIC!
2006
Special Award of the Jury
2015
Best of the Best award by Gourmand, honouring all the books that were awarded Best in the World Over 20 Years

VEGEMANIA
2006
Best Vegetarian Book in the World

HAYLEY'S VEGEMANIA GARDEN
2010
Best Vegetarian Cookbook in Malaysia & Best in the World

HAYLEY'S FRUITASTIC GARDEN
2010
Best Health and Nutrition Book in Malaysia & Best in the World

MYANMAR CUISINE, CULTURE AND CUSTOMS
2014
Best Asian Cuisine Book in the World

HAPPYLICIOUS
2015
Best Food and Family Book in 2016 Malaysia Best Food and Family Book in the World

HAYLEY'S HAPYLICIOUS SERIES
2016
National Winner in its Category: Series
Best Chocolate Book (Individual Category)
Best Fruits Book (Individual Category)

HAYLEY'S VIBRANT VEGETABLES HAYLEY'S FANTASTIC FRUITS
2016
Nautilus Book Awards Silver Winner (Children's Illustrated, Non-Fiction)

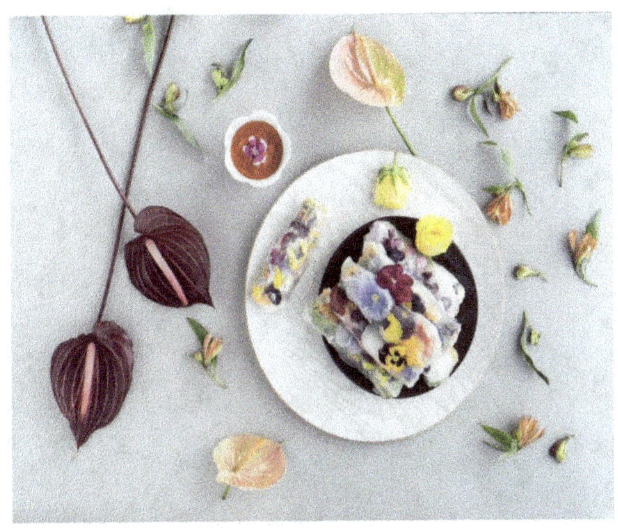

HAYLEY'S FANTASTIC FRUITS
2017
Book Excellence Awards – Finalist
P2P Champion, Pitch-to-Page Competition, Category 1-Idea to Book
Anugerah Buku Negara 2017-Best Of The Best

FLOWERLICIOUS
2019
Gourmand World Cookbook Awards – Best in All (Malaysia) and Top 3 (Natural Health Category)
Book Excellence Awards Finalist
2020
Gourmand World Cookbook Awards – Best in the World winner

HAYLEY'S FANTASTIC FRUITS
2020
IBBY (International Board on Books for Young People) 2020

HAYLEY'S FLOWERLICIOUS MALAYSIA
2020
Gourmand World Cookbook Awards, Best in the World

Spot a title you like? To purchase any of Mohana's books, connect with her at facebook.com/mohana.gill

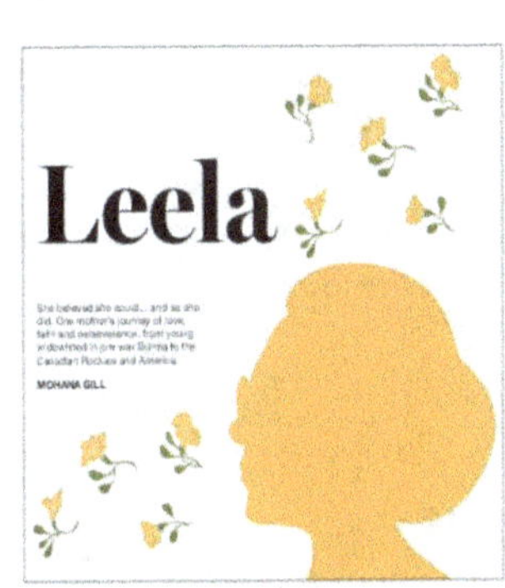

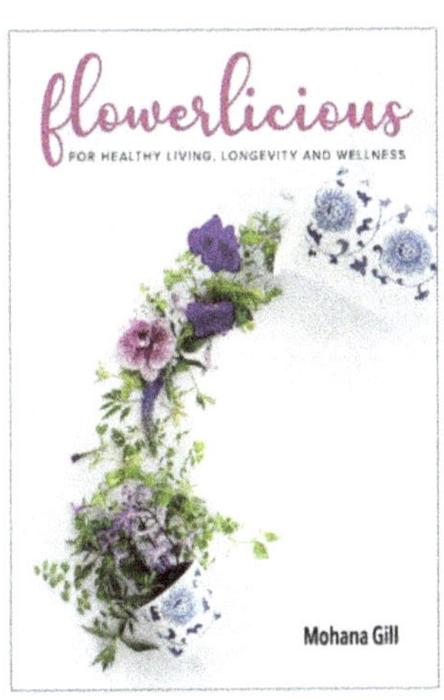

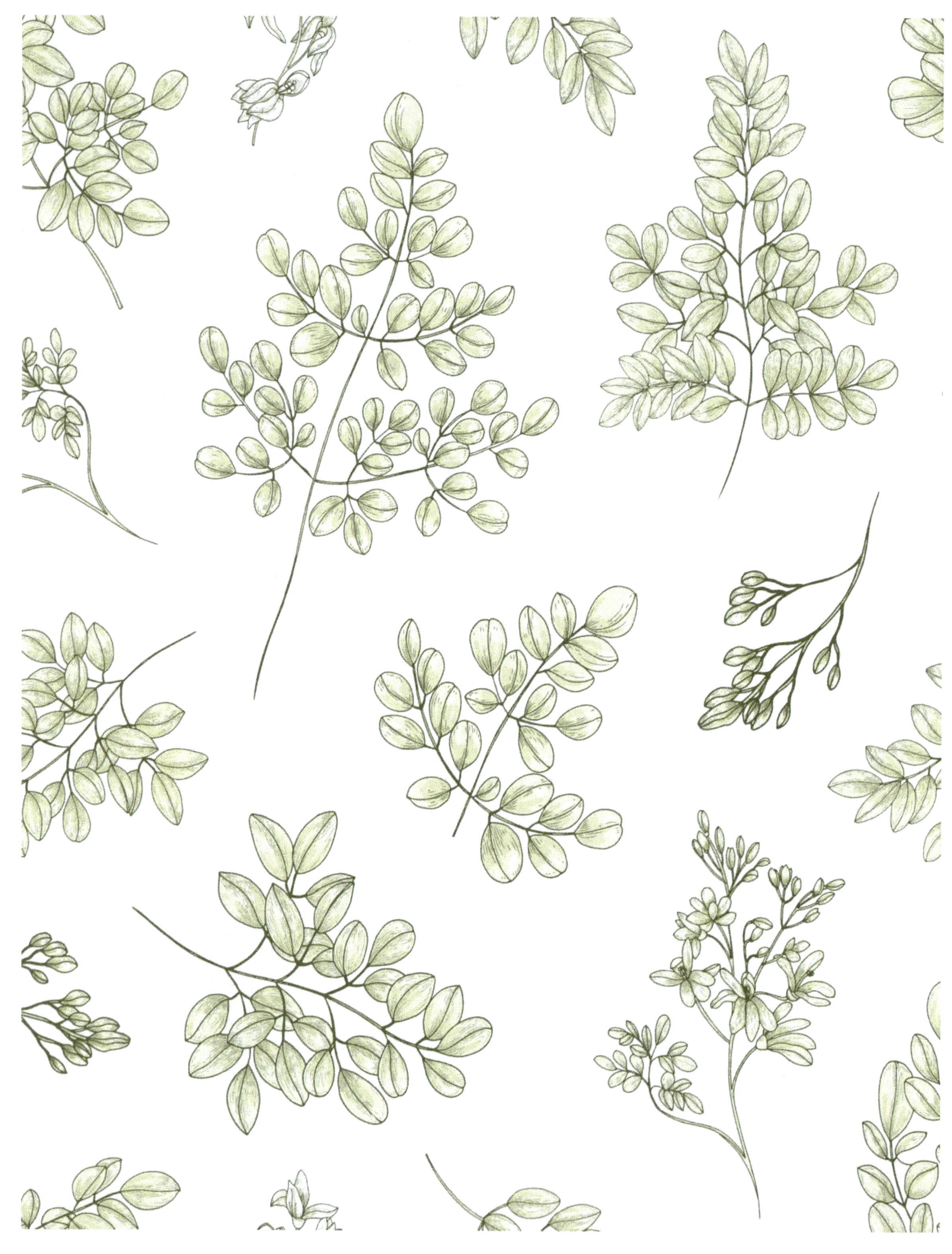

www.ingramcontent.com/pod-product-compliance
Lightning Source LLC
Chambersburg PA
CBHW080938120726
48003CB00011B/3200